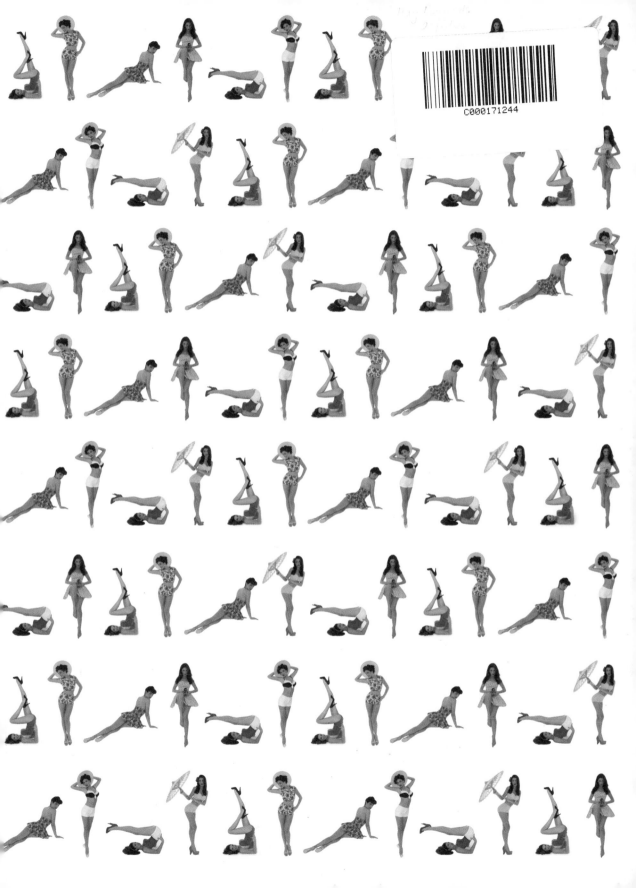

life style

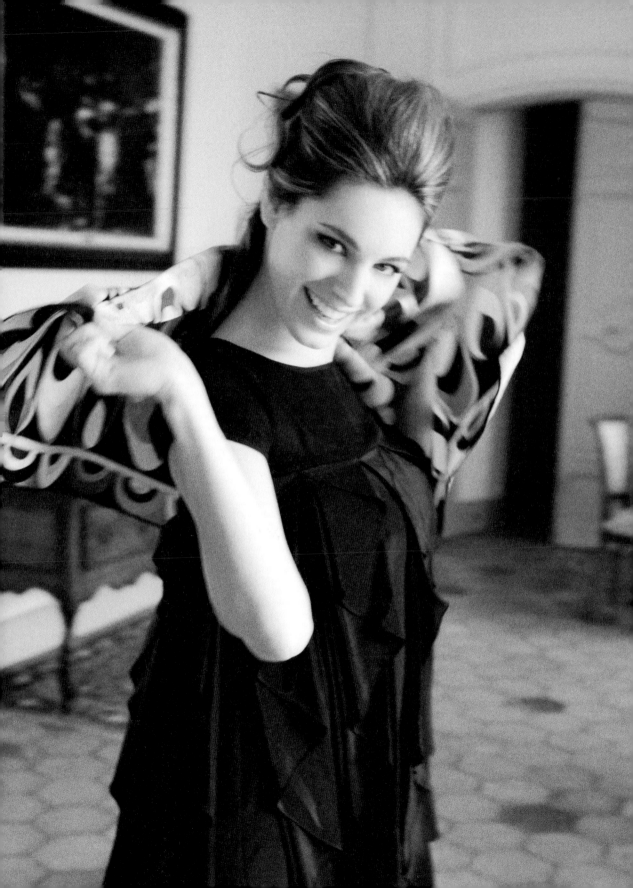

life style

kelly
BROOK

how to pin down the pin-up within you

by Kelly Brook

with Karen Kay

First published in hardback in Great Britain in 2007 by Orion Books
an imprint of the Orion Publishing Group Ltd
Orion House, 5 Upper St Martin's Lane,
London WC2H 9EA
An Hachette Livre UK Company

1 3 5 7 9 10 8 6 4 2

A CIP catalogue record for this book is available
from the British Library.

ISBN: 978 0 7528 8956 6
Printed in Spain by Cayfosa-Quebecor
Design by Smith & Gilmour, London

The Orion Publishing Group's policy is to use papers that are
natural, renewable and recyclable and made from wood grown in
sustainable forests. The logging and manufacturing processes are
expected to conform to the environmental regulations of the
country of origin.

Every effort has been made to fulfil requirements with regard to
reproducing copyright material. The author and publisher will be
glad to rectify any omissions at the earliest opportunity.

www.orionbooks.co.uk

to Tom, Millie, Shannon & Brandon

contents

acknowledgements

So many people have contributed to this book in some way or another and, although I may miss out a few names, I would like to thank the following:

Thank you to Karen Kay for bringing her expertise, honesty and humour to this project. You are a wonderful lady who I wanted to work with before I even knew you were a fashion journalist. I am so pleased that our combined passions, stories and interests created such a great book that I will always be proud to call my first.

I would like to thank Jon Fowler and Ian Marshall for putting up with my obsessive need for everything to be better, and also for allowing the team a wicked trip to the South of France – I know it wasn't in the budget.

Thank you to the 'Glam Squad', Ginny Bogado, Jonathan Malone and Kim Goodwin, for creating so many wonderful looks over the years and never running out of ideas. You are great friends as well as incredible artists.

A special thank you to Dean Freeman, Terri Manduca and the whole photographic team for making my vision become a reality and more. I had so much fun in France, I hope we can do it again soon.

I would also like to thank Alon Shulman, Alan Strutt, Richard Rosenberg, Andrew Ruff, Marc Sniderman, Lewis Kaye, Lin Milano, Joan Hyler, Daniel Galvin Jnr, Alan Dallo, Hakaan Kousetta and Jonathan Hackford.

Without the love and support of my family and friends nothing would be possible, so I would like to take this opportunity to say thank you to my mum and dad. I love you both so much and am so happy that this book has meant I could be home and see you so much more. To my brother Damien and his girlfriend Kelly, thank you for the kids. It buys me a few more years and keeps Mum and Dad quiet. To my sister Sacha, I love you so much and you really are too beautiful for your own good.

The birds, Sadie, Lisa, Jo, Dannielle, Suzie and Susie, my best friends and partners in crime.

And thank you to Billy. You are why I wrote this book, thank you for being my biggest fan. I love you loads, xx.

Again I would like to thank everyone at Orion for making this book such a wonderful experience.

To my fans, thank you for everything. Love and kisses, Kelly Brook

---

Karen Kay would like to thank Ian Marshall, Anna Valentine and the rest of the team at Orion for their dedication to this project, and Shauna Bartlett for being a patient and considerate editor. Thanks, too, to Emma Parry and Kate Scherler for your invaluable advice and expertise when I didn't know where to turn.

Kelly, I've loved working with you every high-heeled, glamour-fuelled step of the way. Your infectious passion for life is filled with an innate sense of style and a wonderful humour and generous spirit, all qualities that have inspired a lasting friendship. I've thoroughly enjoyed the journey we've taken together, and hope that we will continue to share many more laughter-filled moments ahead.

To Dries van Noten, for injecting beauty into my life on a daily basis.

To my parents, Ann and Bill, and my sister, Gayle; my love and thanks for being there, always, through the highs and lows of my life. I am blessed to know how special 'family' really is.

And to Ian, my best friend, lover and life partner. You know me, understand me and love me unconditionally for who I am – including the mountain of shoes. Thank you for supporting and encouraging me throughout this project, when we were nurturing a very special 'project' of our own. Who knows how the next chapter of our life together will unfold, but with you by my side, I know I'll cherish every minute of it…

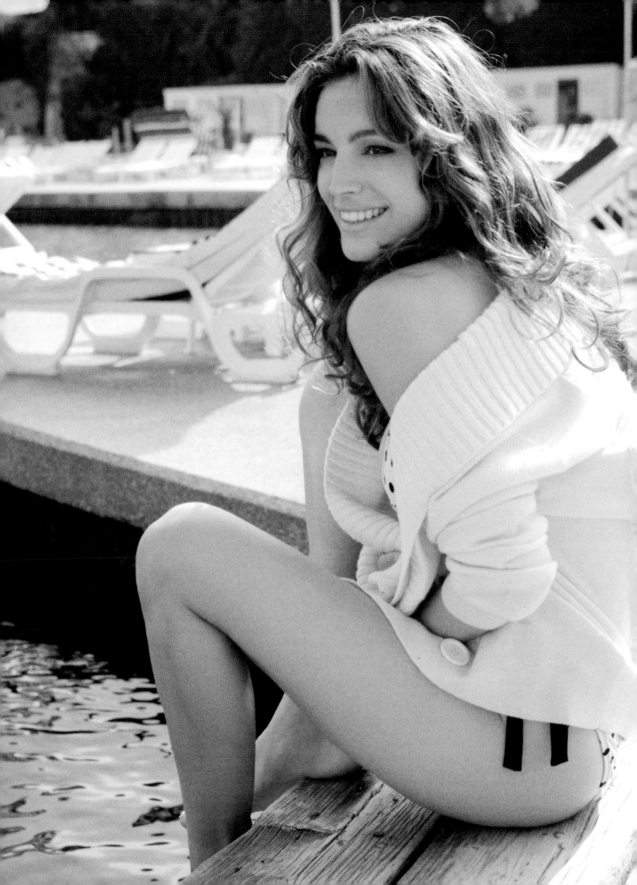

introduction

As far back as I can remember, I have always loved to dress up. When I was just a little girl, I would parade in dresses that my grandmother had made, putting on shows in the playground, and in our living room at home. In these frilly pink or lilac numbers, I would be transported to another world: a place where women were glamorous creatures who wore pretty frocks with cherry-red lipstick and high heels. My fantasy world was a long, long way from the small town where I grew up in Kent, but I never let that deter me: I always aspired to live a more glamorous life.

"I always aspired to live a more glamorous life"

As well as dressing up I adored performing, and I've been lucky enough to combine both of these passions in my career as a model, actress and designer.

I'm fully aware of the irony that I'm writing about style and clothes, though, as when I first made my name I didn't usually wear very much. To me, however, style is about self-awareness and a chic approach to life, rather than fitting a mould or a prescriptive way of dressing.

I honestly believe that a woman can look as stylish and alluring in a bra and briefs or a bikini as she can in a beautiful evening gown on the red carpet. She can be slim or curvy, tall or small, blonde or brunette. It's not about having the right label in your jacket or trying to conform to a fashionable ideal. You don't have to own this season's 'It Bag' to look fabulous; nor do you have to be a skinny size 8 or have the curves of a glamour model.

Neurosis isn't attractive. In fact, when I look at women who have dieted themselves into a miserable state, constantly worrying about how many calories they're consuming, I feel desperately sad, because the essence of their femininity has gone. There's no sparkle in their eyes and they seem to have lost the joy that goes with being a woman. A man doesn't notice a woman's waistline first: he notices her smile or her eyes – if she looks happy, confident and fun, that's what appeals. Ask any red-blooded male what he finds attractive. Just look at Marilyn Monroe: she was the hottest woman on the planet and she was no size zero.

Being stylish is all about confidence, grooming, finding a look that suits you and carrying it off with panache. I've definitely made mistakes along the way, but over the years, I've discovered and refined my sense of taste, learning what works with my body shape and finding the courage to avoid being swayed by the diktats of fashion and sticking to what works for me.

For inspiration, I've looked to other women who've celebrated their femininity, rejoicing in their curves and dressing to enhance their shape. For me, the female ideal is someone who's happy with who they are, and who doesn't feel a need to conform. Who wants to be the sheep that follows every fashion? Far better to stand out as an individual, I say.

In this book I'll be encouraging you to discard the desire to follow the crowd, and instead set out on a voyage of discovery: find out who you are and what makes you feel good when you get dressed in the morning. If certain colours and styles put a smile on your face and attract compliments from others, run with them.

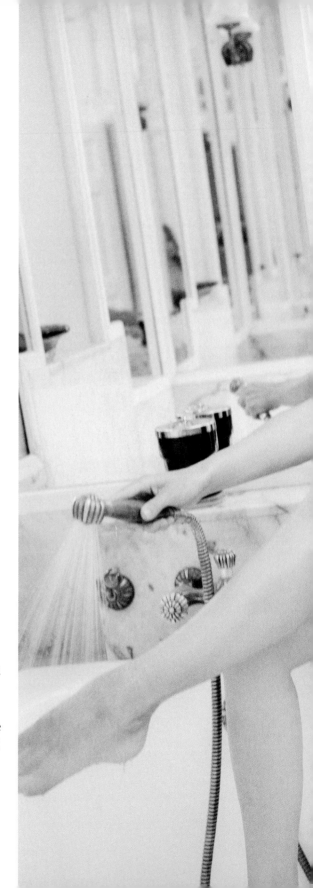

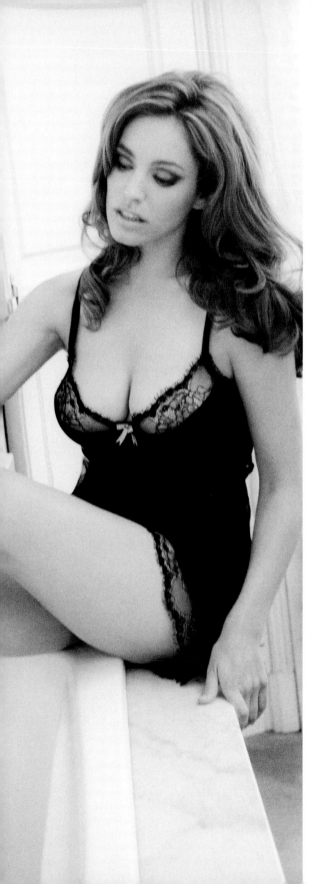

If skinny jeans or miniskirts make you feel uncomfortable, no matter how this season they are, reject them and wear the pieces that put a spring in your step. A lot of looking good is having the confidence to follow your intuition – you know instinctively when something feels good, but it can take time to develop the self-confidence to go against the grain. The trick to finding your fashion feet is not about learning to wear *every* look the glossy magazines promote: it's about knowing when not to wear them!

The aim of this book is to tell the story of how I came to be where I am today, looking at the parts of my childhood and career that have really helped shape my style, including the Hollywood pin-ups who've inspired my look. From the fancy dress costumes I wore in local carnivals to my film wardrobes; from the bikinis I've modelled to the choices I've made on the red carpet, I've developed a look that suits me and makes me happy.

As Quentin Crisp once declared, fashion is 'what you adopt when you don't know who you are'. Only once you're sure of your own identity can you be true to yourself...

Kelly x

my life + my style =

life style

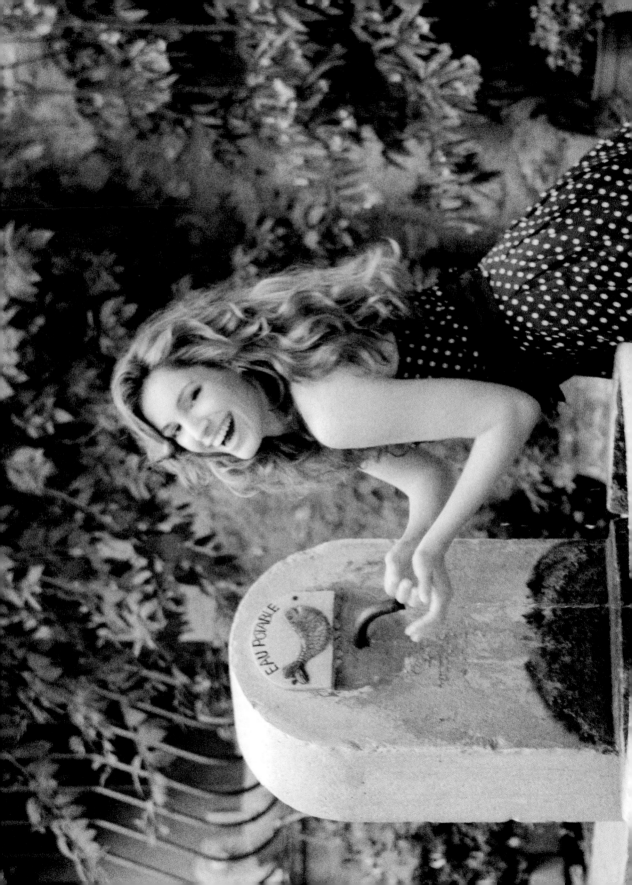

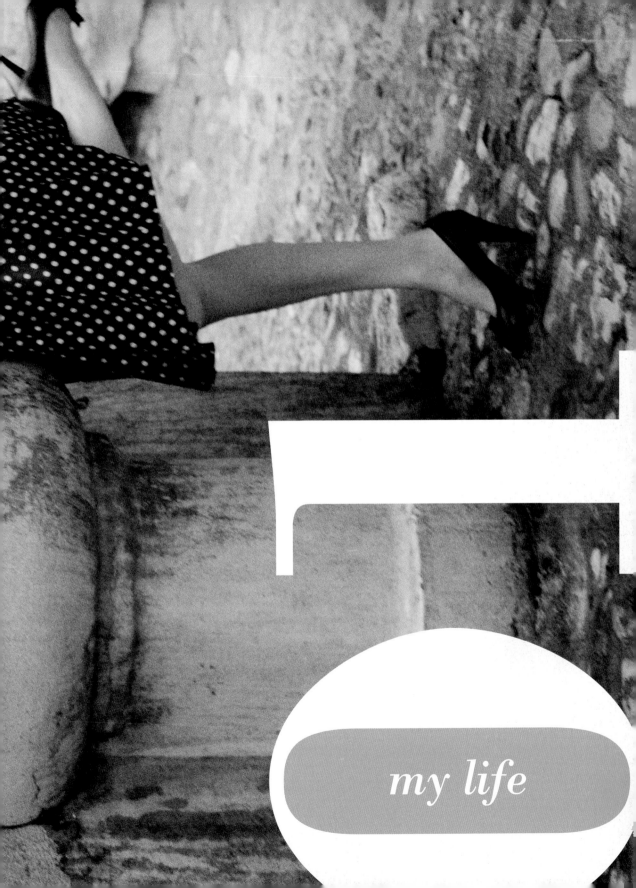

my life

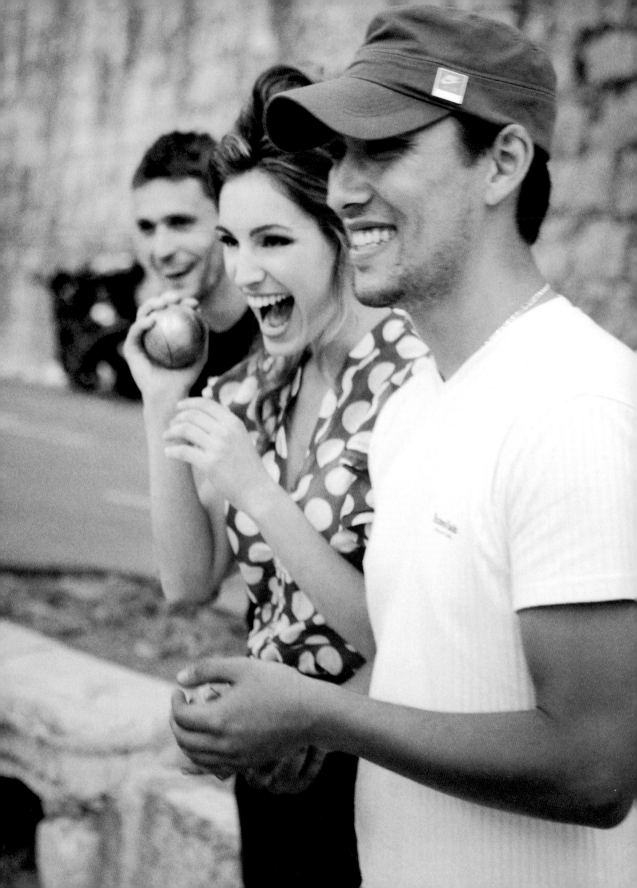

finding my style

It's fitting, when you've spent most of your life daydreaming about being a Hollywood star, to discover that you were nearly named after one of the most glamorous film characters of them all: Scarlett O'Hara. *Gone with the Wind* has always been my mother's favourite movie, and the romantic female lead, played by a young Vivien Leigh, really captured her imagination.

When she gave birth to me, her first child, on 23 November 1979, her instinct was to give me the name of this much-loved silver-screen personality. But in honour of her late brother, who had tragically died at a young age, she called me Kelly, which was her maiden name, to keep the family name alive for another generation.

Sandra Kelly, my mum, met my dad, Kenneth Parsons, when she was still a schoolgirl in Rochester in Kent, as she had been in the same class as his sister. Dad was twenty-nine and had been married before, but they quickly fell in love, and when mum was only seventeen they were married at Chatham Register Office, near my mum's home. He really was her high-school sweetheart!

I arrived not long after: Kelly Ann Parsons, a healthy baby girl, weighing six pounds, ten and a half ounces. Even when I was born I had masses of dark hair, so much so that when my grandfather came to visit in Chatham hospital, he said to Mum, 'I've bought peanuts for your monkey'. Needless to say, she was quite upset.

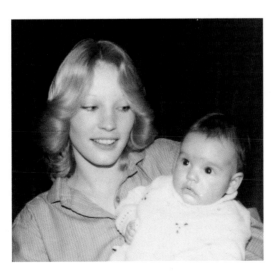

left: With my mum Sandra as a baby.

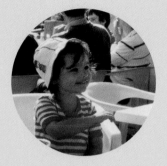
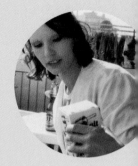

My brother, Damian, came along soon after, and from an early age we got on well and had a happy childhood. My dad worked as a scaffolder and Mum stayed at home to look after the house and raise the family. Mum is a really solid, down-to-earth woman who has always put her family first, and we lived in an average family home in a small city in the south-east of England, and I had a fairly normal suburban Eighties upbringing.

Rochester is incredibly picturesque, with a cobbled high street, a twelfth-century castle – when it was built, the square 113-foot tower was the tallest in England – and a beautiful cathedral which is Britain's second oldest. As children, we grew up celebrating one of our best-known local residents, Charles Dickens, who lived in Rochester and wrote many of his most famous works in the city.

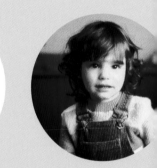

Many of my childhood memories are of playing outside with other kids who lived nearby, many of whom are still close pals now. I loved playing in the garden as a young girl, picking daffodils in the spring and making perfume out of rose petals. We didn't have computers, just the family TV, so much of my time was spent on the local allotments and in orchards, where my friends and I would go scrumping for apples and carrots. There we'd pick raspberries and blackberries from the brambles and make camps. I was very much an outdoor girl and that's still true today – I'm at my happiest in a pair of wellington boots!

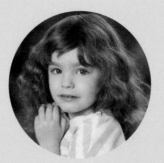

My earliest memories are at the age of
two, when we went on holiday to St Tropez in the
south of France. I have a vivid memory of wearing
dungarees with a red and white stripy T-shirt,
accessorised with a Pinocchio rubber ring that I
insisted on taking everywhere we went. As a toddler,
before I showed an interest in dressing up and girly
clothes, Mum used to put me in practical jersey tops
and dungarees, so I looked like a proper tomboy.

By the age of four I was usually to be found
wearing a white dress with a red cherry print that
my grandmother, Pamela, had bought me. It was
way too big for me and the two triangles of fabric
that were supposed to go over my chest hung much
too low over my midriff, but I refused to take it off,
even at night, because I loved it so much. I screamed
and screamed every morning as Mum tried to dress
me in practical clothes to play in the garden, so that
in the end she had to give in and let me wear the
cherry-print dress.

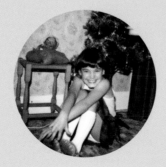

clockwise from top left: On holiday
in my red and white stripy T-shirt in
St Tropez with my mother; smiling
for the camera; enjoying Christmas,
aged seven; as a toddler, I loved
wearing dungarees.

Even as a young girl, I had very definite views on what I wanted to wear, as well as favourite clothes that I demanded to put on in the morning. Nothing's changed there then! That dress has always remained a favourite, as it's associated with all the happy times I had as a child. Even now cherry prints always bring a smile to my face, so when I designed my swimwear collection recently, I insisted on getting a fun cherry design in there.

below: My grandmother and grandfather at King's House in Kuala Lumpur, Malaya, in 1956. My grandfather had just been awarded a British Empire Medal for services to Queen and country.

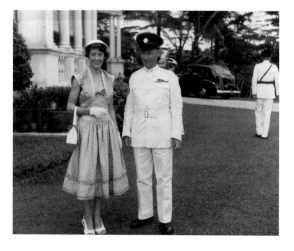

My maternal grandmother, Ann Kelly, who I know as Granny Kelly, was also a huge influence on my early style. When I was small, there was a photograph of her in our living room which, to me, epitomised everything that was ladylike and elegant.

Granny and Grandpa Kelly lived in Malaya for many years, and as a child I was entranced by a particular picture, taken at King's House (the Malayan Prime Minister's house) in Kuala Lumpur in 1956. Granny Kelly was wearing a pale dove-grey spotted cotton organdie full-skirted dress with a matching bolero jacket and a neat little white hat. Her hands were clad in white cotton gloves, she wore white peep-toed slingback heels and carried a small structured white bag on her arm. My grandfather looked so handsome in his starched white uniform and they complemented each other perfectly. To this day I think it's wonderful when couples' dress styles complement each other.

Granny Kelly was an incredibly talented seamstress, and would regularly take me shopping to the local haberdasher's after school to buy material so she could make me a new dress. I seem to remember being rather vocal about my choice of fabrics, too. She taught me to sew, and I've been knitting since I was little – I find it really relaxing and often knit during downtime when I'm on set.

My mum has always been a needlewoman as well, and makes booties, blankets and all sorts of cute little presents for my nieces and nephews. I can remember sitting with her as we sewed mini outfits for my Barbie doll, who was one of my treasured possessions at the time.

Every year, Granny Kelly would spend weeks making a really special dress for me to wear to the Dickens Festival that's staged every summer in Rochester in honour of our local literary hero. Her costume-making was a long, labour-intensive process – and it was probably quite stressful, dressing the little diva that I was then.

My first Dickens Festival appearance, walking in the procession – as I got older, I danced and sang songs from musicals, performing on the high street with a local theatre company – led to my newspaper debut – on the front page of the *Medway Standard*. Even at the tender age of two I was making the news! I wore a little floral pinafore with a matching bonnet, courtesy of Granny Kelly, of course, and it was the first of many wonderful creations.

From about the age of six, my best friend Lisa, who'd moved in a few doors down from us, would enter the festival with me, and together we'd plan our outfits with military precision. I had a chimney sweep costume one year, and all sorts of other period ensembles, each handmade to perfection by my wonderful grandmother. Granny Kelly is still a nimble needlewoman today: just last Christmas, to celebrate my move into a farmhouse in Kent, she knitted me a complete nativity set, complete with loads of animals and a stable.

One of the most beautiful costumes she made was in 1990: it was a lavender satin dress, edged in delicate white lace, and it must have taken her hours and hours. She made me a matching lace parasol, frilly white bloomers and a huge lavender and white bonnet, then she bought me some cute little black patent ankle boots and white lace gloves. When I put the complete outfit on for the first time, I felt utterly fabulous. That year, I was awarded the 'Best Dressed' prize, and I can still remember the moment when they called out my name – I felt all tingly inside, I was so proud!

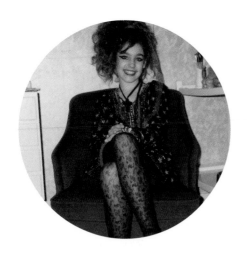

My childhood nickname had been Smelly Parsnips – a childish play on Kelly Parsons – and I was quite a goofy kid. One day around that time we were at an amusement park in Margate when Goofy walked past and my dad said, 'Oh, look, there's Kelly!' My mum was really upset about it and hated it so she marched me off to the dentist to get me a brace. However, as I was only eleven, the dentist said it was too early as my jaw was still developing, but Mum didn't want me to have to wear a brace as a teenager.

I've always adored dressing up, and as a child I loved pretty colours, girly prints and feminine dresses. While my girlfriends were running around in jeans and trainers, I liked nothing more than a few ruffles.

I had a bit of a thing for ra-ra skirts too: I was obsessed with polka-dot ones and thought the frills were wonderfully frivolous. That was one fashion trend I followed with a vengeance. At Christmas, Mum would buy me sparkly tights from Tammy Girl to wear with my ra-ra skirt – I thought I was the bee's knees in my 'grown-up' clothes. It made me feel like Madonna in the 'La Isla Bonita' video, which at that point in my life seemed the height of cool.

I worshipped at the altar of Madonna for a number of years, and my friends and I used to copy a few of her looks. From the lace fingerless gloves to the rag-curled hair and lacy footless tights, I've been there and done it all. If I could have got away with it, I would have worn crucifixes, lacy lingerie, leggings, eyeliner and backcombed hair every day.

"I've always enjoyed dressing up"

Lisa and I also loved Bros, led by a pair of brothers – Luke and Matt Goss – who were huge in the late Eighties and early Nineties. We had posters of them on our bedroom walls and would strap bottle tops to our shoes, religiously following a trend that they started. And my childhood idols were to make a strange reappearance in my life much later on.

For my partner Billy's fortieth birthday in February 2006, I hosted a surprise party at the Silent Movie Theatre in Hollywood, where they show Buster Keaton and Charlie Chaplin movies. His sister, Lisa, who's a jazz singer, performed and I did a 1920s cabaret-style tap dance on stage. A friend of mine, who's a Hollywood agent, brought along a date and introduced us just as I was about to go on stage. It was none other than Luke Goss!

I was mortified to be introduced to the man who used to be pinned on my bedroom wall.

When I was younger, I wasn't allowed to grow my hair beyond shoulder length and always had a fringe, but I used to pull it in a desperate attempt to make it grow. Mum said it would be better if I kept it manageable, but once I was old enough to decide for myself, I let it grow as long as I could. So desperate were my friends to grow their hair that as young teenagers we would all get together before a party and lay my friend Katy on the ironing board, cover her hair with a wet cloth and iron her hair so it was steaming and poker-straight. She used to ask what the awful smell was – in fact, her hair was permed, so it was probably the chemicals burning. It was really stupid, and quite dangerous, looking back on it, but such are the dangers of following fashion too closely.

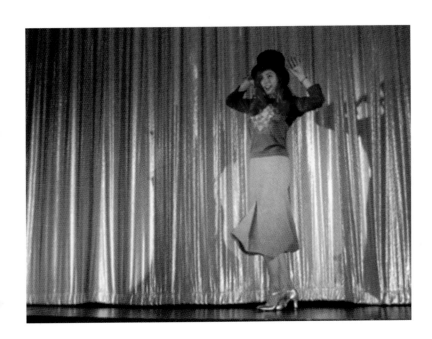

left: On stage performing a tap dance at the Silent Movie Theatre in Hollywood for Billy's fortieth birthday.

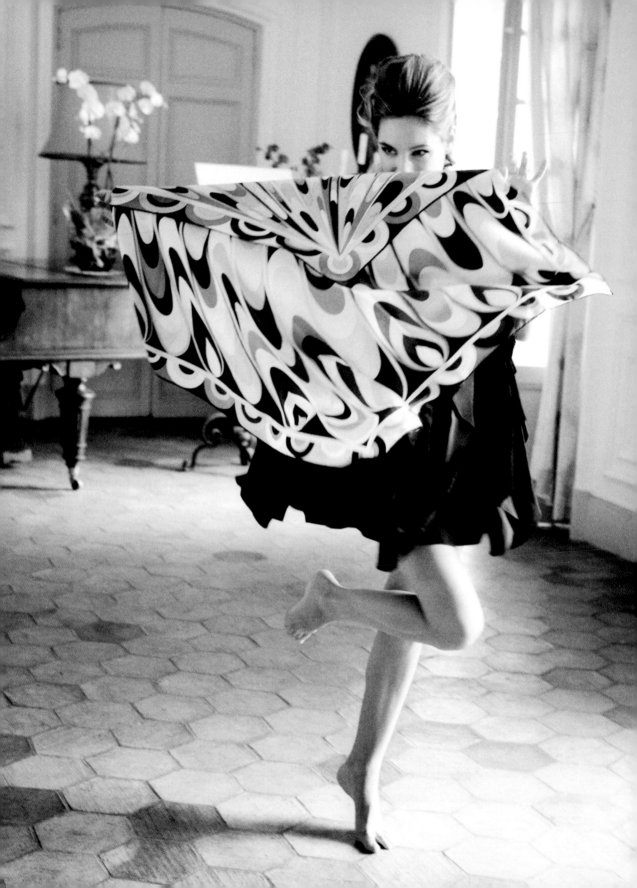

model inspiration

Dad had a daughter, Sacha, by his first wife, who was ten when I was born, and when I was growing up I used to idolise her. She lived with her grandmother, but we saw quite a lot of her and she used to wear really cool clothes that I desperately wanted to try on. She signed with Models 1 in her teens, and suddenly she began appearing in shop windows, on billboards and in magazines. I thought she was so glamorous, modelling in campaigns for Marks & Spencer. Can you imagine how strange it was seeing my sister on posters in local shops? I used to collect her magazine cuttings and even pinched a couple of the posters she appeared on so I could put them up in my bedroom at home.

By the time I was eight or nine, Sacha was – as far as I was concerned, at least – the coolest person on the planet. She had an amazing wardrobe and even had her belly button pierced. She was 5 foot 10, with punky, cropped hair, and seemed to be living a life that was a million miles from the one we knew.

One day she arrived at our house with a new boyfriend, who turned out to be the pop singer,

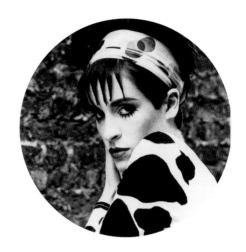

Seal, who's now supermodel Heidi Klum's partner. My friends and I were completely overwhelmed with excitement – my sister was dating a rock star! News spread around school like wildfire, and everyone wanted to know the details. Of course, I didn't know anything, being an innocent younger sibling. They did, however, take me and my brother to Margate for the day, and then we saw pictures of them together in the newspapers. It was my first taste of celebrity!

Sometimes, at weekends, I was allowed to go and stay with her in London, which made me the envy of all my friends. In the school holidays, she would take me along to castings, where I'd sit around waiting for ages, watching all the girls traipse in and out of the studios. My strongest memory of those days is one of extreme hunger: I don't think Sacha ate very much and I didn't want to be a pain by moaning that I was starving.

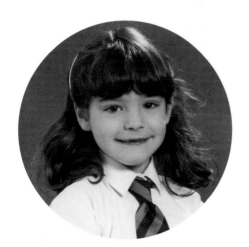

left: I always wanted long hair but had a bob with a bad fringe! **above:** Sacha in a fashion shoot in the 1980s.

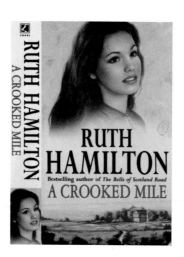

A few years later, when I was about twelve, I remember telling Sacha I was a passionate Betty Boo fan, and she asked her friend Meg Matthews – yes, Noel Gallagher's ex – to get her autograph for me. It meant so much to me at the time and I couldn't wait to show it to my mum and dad. I will always remember how important that was to me as a youngster: it's easy to be dismissive of kids who want an autograph, but it means an awful lot if you stop and sign something for them. If I can make someone feel good just by writing my name, why not do it?

Though I thought Sacha's lifestyle was unbelievably glamorous, I never aspired to be a model. I loved performing, so the thought of sitting still and having my picture taken just didn't appeal, even though my mother and grandmother were keen for me to give it a try. So Mum put me on the books of a junior modelling agency when I was eleven, and I did a few small jobs, including posing for an artist who was illustrating book covers. He did *The Enchanted Castle* by E. Nesbitt, and I still have a copy of the novel I appeared on – *A Crooked Mile*, by Ruth Hamilton – but somehow it doesn't feel like me in the picture, as I just wasn't comfortable with the whole modelling thing. It felt too strange, posing just to look pretty.

At thirteen Mum entered me into a beauty pageant without my knowledge. She sent the local newspaper a photograph with a poem that said 'To be a carnival princess would be the best, I would love to parade in a beautiful dress.' When the phone call came to tell us I'd won, I was gobsmacked. A photographer from the paper took me to a poppy field where I did my first cover shoot, and the pictures appeared on the front page of the *Medway News*. I was extremely embarrassed when all my friends had copies at school.

Soon after, I was paraded through Rochester in a beautiful vintage Rolls-Royce as Carnival Queen. I rather enjoyed the experience, as we led the parade, taking a tour around the town that culminated in an afternoon tea ceremony in Chatham Dockyard. Oh, the glamour!

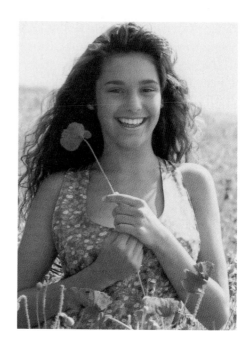

" to be a carnival princess would be the best, I would love to parade in a beautiful dress **"**

drama queen to model student

Though I wasn't entirely at ease modelling, I did enjoy performing: I loved dancing and acting and was always putting on little shows in our living room at home, demanding that Mum, Dad and Damian sit and watch my new routines. I used to stage mini productions in the school playground with my friends, so you can see that I enjoyed being the centre of attention!

When I was ten or eleven, I went to see a fortune teller on Margate Pier as I wanted to know what I would be when I grew up. I'd always believed I would be an actress, and she told me I wouldn't have to try hard and that I should just be myself and things would come to me, which seemed strange as I was always acting out roles as other people.

A big influence on my style as a child was the TV series, *Fame*, starring Irene Cara. It was all about life in a New York performing arts school, and I used to beg my mum to let me watch it, then I'd learn all the words to the songs and copy all the dance moves. I would prance around the house, doing star jumps off the sofa and singing the soundtrack – 'Fame! I wanna live for ever! I wanna learn how to fly!' – at the top of my voice.

On one occasion, I did a straddle jump from the sofa and completely misjudged it: I ended up in hospital having butterfly stitches to mend the cut above my left eye. I still have a scar to this day – that'll teach me to try and be Leroy!

By the time I was twelve, I was desperate to go to a school like the one in *Fame*. I wanted to be an actress and a star. I loved the idea of being famous. I was a pupil at a big, modern comprehensive called Thomas Aveling School in Rochester at the time, with loads of friends who I loved, but I still had an overwhelming desire to go to stage school. Nothing in the standard curriculum inspired me and I had an irrepressible urge to perform.

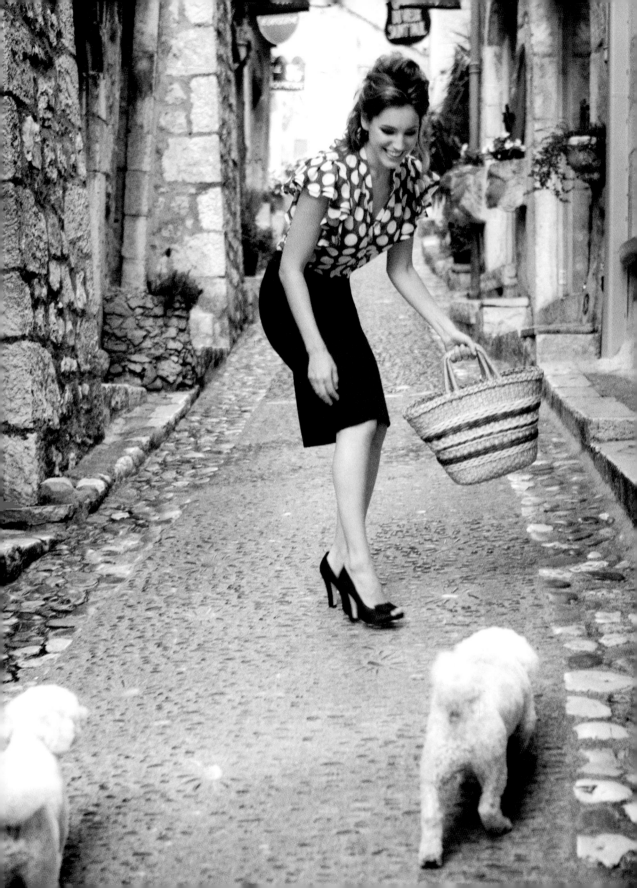

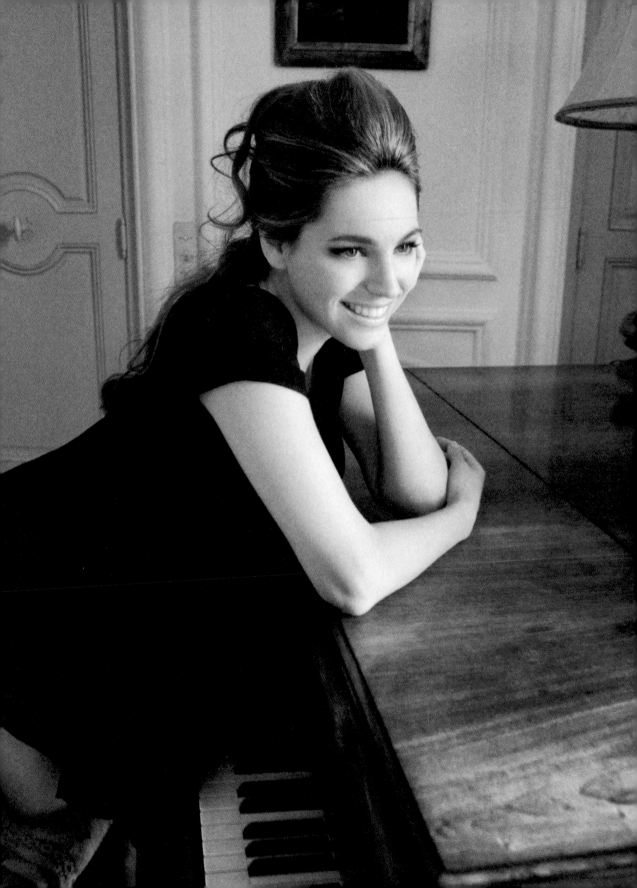

I began asking my mother to send me
to stage school, and after months of incessant
begging and pleading, she finally agreed to write
to the Italia Conti Academy of Theatre Arts, near
the Barbican in London. They sent us a prospectus,
and it was everything I'd ever dreamed of: Italia
Conti is Britain's oldest performing arts school
and has been going since 1911. As well as studying
regular school curriculum subjects such as maths,
science, French, history, etc., pupils learn ballet, tap,
modern and jazz dance, musical theatre, acting and
singing, in preparation for becoming 'leaders of the
entertainment industry of tomorrow'. Needless to
say, I was more determined than ever to make my
dream a reality.

Some of Italia Conti's famous alumni

Noel Coward
Sadie Frost
Claire Goose
Olivia Hussey
Letitia Dean
Naomi Campbell
Leslie Ash
Bonnie Langford
Emily Lloyd
Millicent Martin
Martine McCutcheon
Anthony Newley
Nanette Newman
Sharon Osbourne
Leslie Phillips
Jenny Powell
Louise Redknapp
Nadia Sawalha
Julia Sawalha
Dinah Sheridan
Lisa Snowdon
Claire Sweeney
Tracey Ullman
Lena Zavaroni

And of course ... Kelly Brook

For the audition, I had to prepare a tap dance, ballet dance and jazz dance, then perform two set acting pieces and sing a song. After six weeks of extra Saturday classes in Rochester I felt ready, but I was still a bag of nerves when Mum and I took the train to London for the audition. Despite the butter-flies in my stomach, I managed to perform my dance routines really well, and was very pleased with the way the acting and singing went, too. As we made our way home on the train, through the suburbs of south-east London, I knew I'd given it my best shot, which, after all, is all anyone can do.

The head teacher had told us we'd receive a letter within a week, informing us whether I had won a place or not, so I spent the following days in a state of flux. I tried to take my mind off things, desperately convincing myself that there was nothing more

I could do to influence the decision, but I couldn't concentrate at school and lay awake at night wondering if the postman would bring the letter the next morning.

Eventually, after what seemed like a lifetime, though was actually only seven days, as the school had promised, the envelope arrived. As I slid my finger along the top, splitting it open, I felt the butterflies again in my belly. Thankfully, the news was positive: I'd secured a place at stage school. I danced around the kitchen, hugging my mum and dad.

Though I was going to be very sad to leave my schoolfriends, I knew I was incredibly lucky to have this once-in-a-lifetime opportunity, and I was filled with excitement at the prospect of starting.

One of the first things we had to do was buy my new uniform: Mum was horrified that the only place that sold the official school kit was Harrods. I was to wear a light blue kilt, a white cotton shirt embroi-dered with the pale blue school emblem and a dark blue blazer. No popping into the local M&S for a standard-issue skirt and shirt! We had a two-hour train journey to get there, and when we saw the prices, we decided to buy everything big so it would last as long as possible.

'Oh my God, Kelly,' moaned Mum, as we travelled home from Knightsbridge laden with green and gold shopping bags. 'Only you would want to attend a school where the uniform has to come from Harrods.'

When I was invited back to Harrods in 2006 to open their January sale, I had a quiet giggle to myself when Billy and I, escorted by Mohamed Al Fayed plus bagpipers and photographers, walked past the section where I'd had my uniform fitted all those years earlier. It was worth it, after all, Mum.

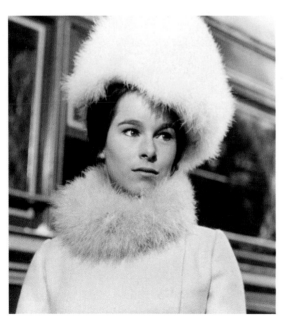

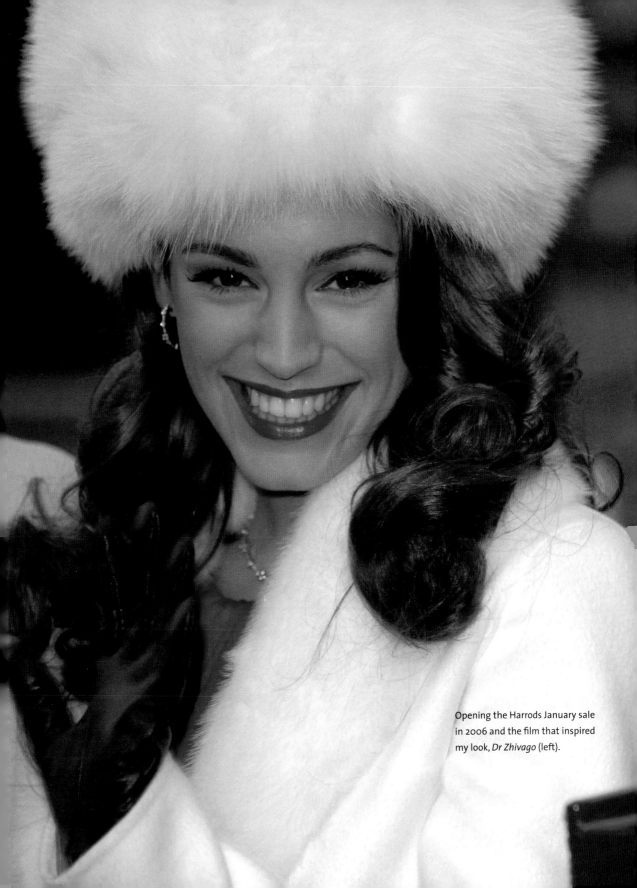

Opening the Harrods January sale
in 2006 and the film that inspired
my look, *Dr Zhivago* (left).

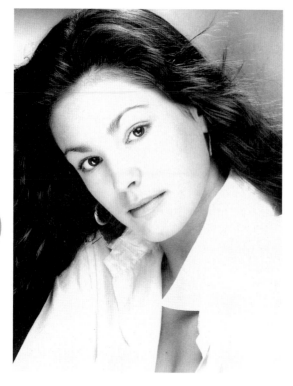

above: My first professional headshot for Italia Conti at the age of fourteen.

Even as a fourteen-year-old, I realised that Mum and Dad were making a lot of sacrifices to send me to Italia Conti, and that I was extremely lucky they were willing to indulge my fantasies. It was my determination but their money, and it cost them a fortune. That's something I'll always be grateful for.

In January 1994, I started at Italia Conti, news that was reported in the *Medway News*, who quoted me as their former carnival queen: 'I have wanted to be a star ever since I was a child. But it was the winning of the carnival princess title that gave me the boost of confidence I needed to really go for it.'

That was my first experience of being misquoted in the press – these days, you have to laugh it off when you read things you've supposedly said and haven't.

The day before I was due to start at my new school, my mum decided to tackle my 'mono-brow'. I've always had a prolific head of hair, which is often the envy of other women. I know I'm really lucky, but the downside is that it's often accompanied by bushy eyebrows – remember Brooke Shields? – and mine had grown into one big brow that dominated my forehead.

Mum pinned me down and numbed my skin with ice cubes before plucking away at the dark hairs that were surplus to requirement. I screamed in pain – the ice cubes didn't exactly have the same effect as local anaesthetic – but I also remember laughing hysterically as my mum attacked me with the tweezers.

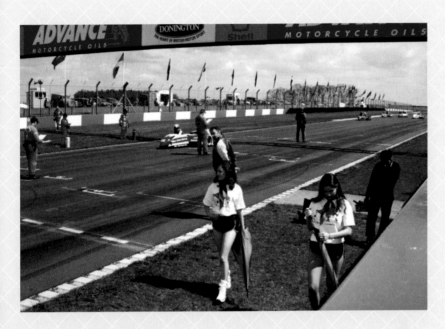

On my first day, the one thing I remember is that all the girls had skirts down to the floor, while mine was knee length with growing room at the waist. My friend Danielle still recalls how wrong I got it: even school uniforms have an unwritten look.

Aside from Danielle, however, I think most of the girls spent more time looking at my eyebrows, as the next day everyone had tried to copy my neatly plucked shape. Unfortunately, some went a bit overboard, so there were a few that looked like tadpoles.

Commuting into London on a daily basis was quite a shock for someone used to going to school around the corner: I left home at 6.30 and was on the train each morning by 7 a.m. Another Italia Conti girl, Natasha Green, lived two stops down the line from me, and in the early days she would lean out of the train so my mum could hand me over and we would travel down to London together to be in school for a nine o'clock ballet class. Some days I left even earlier so I could swim at the Barbican pool before school, and most days I'd eventually arrive home at about 7.30 p.m. for dinner, then homework.

I was always exhausted, but I loved it so much that it was worth it. My new routine made me grow up quite quickly, though. For someone who had only been into the city a handful of times, it was a shock to find myself travelling alone with a train full of city commuters every day, and it did wonders for my self-confidence.

At Easter, and sometimes over the Christmas holidays, our family would go to Belgium to stay with my mum's sister, Patricia Kelly, who worked as Senior International Correspondent for CNN, the American TV news channel, which is based in Brussels. When I was younger, we rode bikes and played on their farm just outside the city, where they had chickens and geese. My aunt would stage fabulous Easter egg hunts, hiding treats all around the farm, and it would keep us occupied for hours. It was definitely worth the effort as the chocolate, as you'd expect in Belgium, was to die for!

I remember how, whenever she was due to appear on TV, we would all gather round and watch her in her bullet-proof vest and helmet, reporting from Sarajevo, Kosovo or wherever she happened to be at the time.

Just like my model sister Sacha, Aunty Patsy was up there on a pedestal for me, as someone really inspirational – my interest in broadcasting stemmed from a visit to the CNN studios in Brussels at the age of twelve; it was a real eye-opener to the awe-inspiring world of live television. I was bowled over by what a powerful medium it could be, potentially

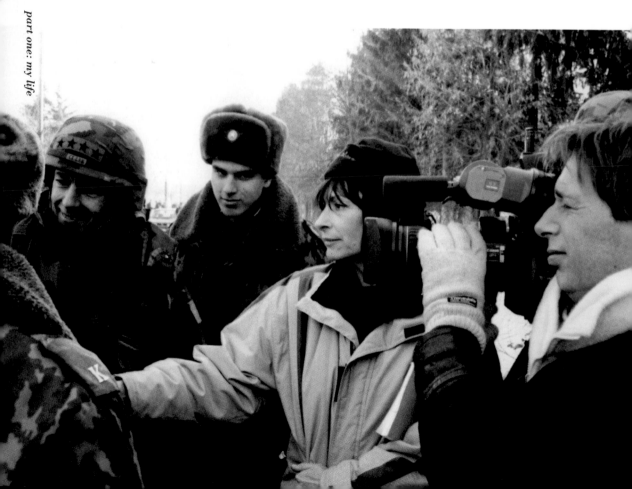

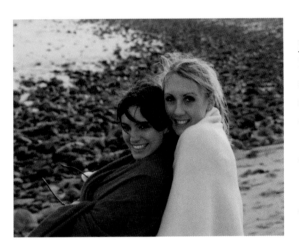

For a while, I considered becoming a journalist, but as I explored different forms of media, I realised there wasn't much difference between my aunt and Steven Spielberg: they're both storytellers, shedding light and information on important topics and using their medium as a form of communication.

Though I loved my Media Studies course, and adored all the dance and acting classes, I also loved art and had an amazing art teacher called Miss Todd, who was against the idea of us having to wear school uniform. She believed that as theatre students, we were obliged to be more creative with our wardrobes than 'normal' school pupils. She honestly felt we should be encouraged to express our individuality and creativity in every way possible, and eventually persuaded our headmaster to let us wear our own clothes on Fridays. Needless to say, we were over the moon.

influencing an audience's view on politics, religion, war and all sorts of subjects.

This fascination led me to take Media Studies a year early at school, where I learned about Russian propaganda and the innovative film-maker Serge Eisenstein. I began to understand how there was a big crossover between what was deemed entertainment and what was considered factual broadcasting, and became a big fan of European movies as a result. I like the way they stimulate debate and tell stories in a way that's both entertaining and socially influential.

At the time, my friend Lisa and I were obsessed with the 'Crazy' music video by Aerosmith that played on rotation on MTV. It featured Alicia Silverstone and Liv Tyler – the daughter of lead singer Steve Tyler – sneaking out of school and driving through California in a cool convertible car, picking up a cute farm boy on the way. Liv wore a fantastic pair of skin-tight leather trousers, which I coveted more than anything in the world, so for my fifteenth birthday I bought a pair. I thought they were the coolest trousers ever – now all I needed was a ticket to Hollywood!

left: My aunt, the CNN correspondent Patricia Kelly, pictured here with the Russian Army on Christmas Eve 1999. She inspired me to get into broadcasting.

above: 'Crazy girls'. We made it! My childhood friend, Lisa, and me in Malibu, California.

The school had an agency arm, so pupils would be put forward for auditions. There were a wide range of opportunities, and I acted in a drama for the BBC and a couple of TV commercials, but the focus was on completing the school curriculum, not disappearing off to a film location or theatre all the time. That didn't stop the excitement when your name appeared on the school noticeboard, with a request to go and see the agency, though.

Outside school, I had a fairly solid work ethic, and got myself a couple of part-time jobs to earn some pocket money. My father, who worked really hard as a self-employed scaffolding contractor, had instilled the importance of hard work in me, showing that it brought its own rewards.

My weekend job was in an ice cream and cake shop called Precinct Pantry, which was located on a pretty cobbled street next to Rochester Cathedral, overlooking the castle and next to a boys' boarding school. I used to make delicious ice cream, fudge and cakes, and though most of my friends earned more in their jobs, I loved working in the pretty tearoom. I still have a sweet tooth to this day, and can't resist indulging in a pastel-iced cupcake in a beautiful teashop – it's a delightfully girly ritual and my favourite is Red Velvet.

As I was a good dancer, during school holidays and at weekends I would often appear in pantomime or cabaret shows for a company called Hammond Productions, and though the money wasn't great, we had a lot of fun.

Like all teenagers, I was a bit of a brat at times, and when my mum tried to discipline me, I used to shout back at her that she'd regret being nasty to me, because when I was a Hollywood star

below: After baking by day in a cake shop, my weekend job involved dancing at night in a cabaret act.

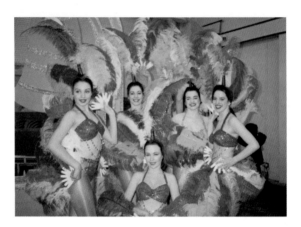

with a big swimming pool I wouldn't take her calls or invite her to lounge with a cocktail with me. I was joking of course, but they do say be careful what you wish for – Mum constantly reminds me of my threats today, on those occasions when we get the chance to sit by the pool enjoying chillout time together.

Soon after I turned sixteen, my mum – again, without telling me – sent my school headshots into a competition to model for amateur photographers. I won and the prize was a modelling assignment in Portugal with a local photographer called Mike Golsby, shooting pictures for a calendar. I didn't tell anyone at school about it, but once again, I ended up being featured in the local paper, who invited me down to a nearby marina to take some shots of me on a boat. I wore a red bikini and the pictures appeared on the cover.

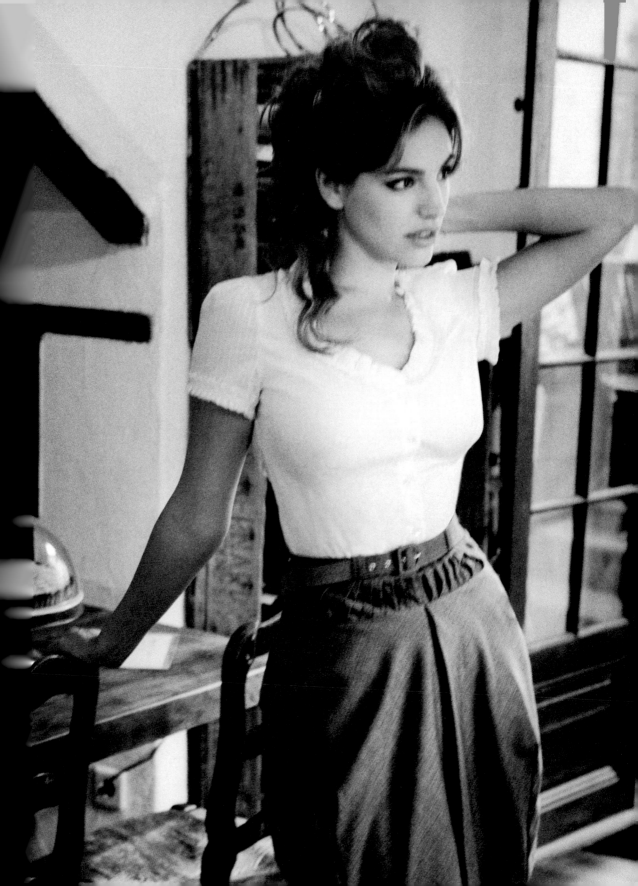

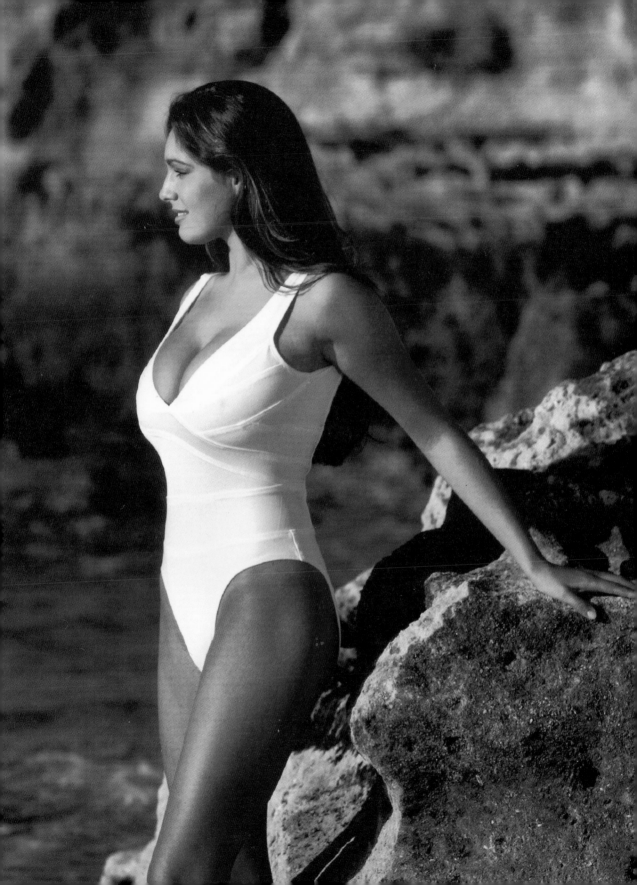

I really enjoyed the shoot in Portugal. I stayed in a lovely rustic house in the hills with four other models, and came home feeling quite positive about doing more glamour modelling work. At 5 foot 6 inches and with a 36E bust, I was too big up top to sign with a fashion modelling agency like my sister.

In fact my boobs started growing when I was eleven and by the time I was thirteen, I was a C cup. I can remember my mum taking me to M&S to buy my first bra, and the woman measured me, then handed me a huge, hideously clumsy thing. All my friends were in delicate little broderie anglaise cotton garments, and I had to wear something our grannies would wear! Despite the fact that I developed so early, I have no idea where my curves come from: my mum has a slender, androgynous frame, like Kate Moss.

In my early days at Italia Conti, I was never self-conscious about my shape, even though my figure wasn't the ideal lean dancer's physique. We spent most of the day looking in the mirror during dance rehersals, so you had no choice but to love what you saw – the girls that didn't were miserable, with even some of the size zeroes not being happy with their bodies. We spent so much of our school day in a leotard and tights that I became comfortable with my shape – you really have no choice as you're not quite as hidden as you are in a skirt, shirt and sweater.

I was encouraged by some of the models I'd met in Portugal to go and see their agent, Samantha Bond, who specialised in glamour work and represented most of the topless models who appeared in Britain's tabloid newspapers at the time.

Samantha was lovely and took me on immediately, agreeing only to put me forward for straightforward glamour work that wasn't too risqué, as I was still at school doing my exams. I was way too shy to do topless work anyway.

left: Having won the beauty contest I was sent to Portugal to model for a swimwear brand called Laura Jane.

I began modelling for catalogues and appeared in some pop videos as well as making some commercials. It was during this time that I learned some of the tricks of the trade when it comes to modelling lingerie and swimwear that I discuss later on in the book. I travelled all over Europe to beautiful locations, including Cyprus, Monaco, Vienna, Madrid, Santorini, Portugal and Venice. I didn't really choose it, it chose me, but I certainly got paid well for doing it, and I loved the travelling that was often involved.

A couple of years after I left Italia Conti, my former headmaster apparently caught some of the boys who were a few years below me at school looking at one of my lingerie layouts in a magazine. I heard that he called the whole school into a special assembly and used the said feature as an example of the path not to take in life.

A while later, soon after I'd landed my job as co-presenter on *The Big Breakfast*, I decided to drop into Italia Conti and say hello to my teachers. The headmaster couldn't have been more pleased to see me, and accompanied me on a school tour, talking to all the pupils about my success in hosting one of television's most popular shows. I didn't mention the assembly he'd called a couple of years earlier, but I was all too aware of the sweet irony of him showing me off to his students.

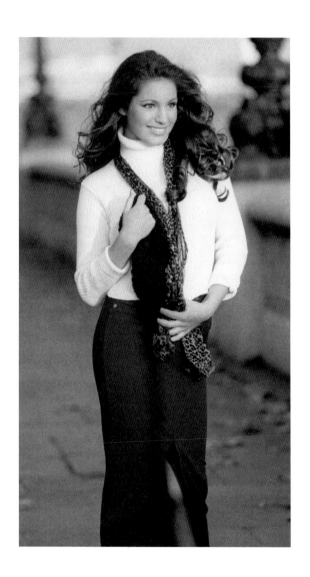

"*the headmaster said I was an example of the path NOT to take*"

new model army

Thanks to my new-found success as a model, loads of other opportunities opened up for me, and one of the most exciting experiences – and something I was really passionate about – was a a trip I made in December 1997 with Joanne Guest, then a very successful glamour model, to Bosnia on a morale-raising mission for the British troops stationed there.

Some of my ancestors were in the armed forces – my great-great-grandfather on my mother's side, Edmund Edward Kelly, signed up to the Royal Navy three days after he turned fifteen, in 1870, and served a total of twenty-four years on fifteen different ships, rising through the ranks from cabin boy to Chief Petty Officer. His son, Ernest Kelly, also joined up at the tender age of fifteen, becoming a sergeant with the Royal Garrison Artillery. He married his sweetheart Bertha when he was twenty-nine, and the couple moved to India, where he was posted soon after the wedding. Ernest and Bertha's only child was Arthur, my grandfather, who served as a staff sergeant with the Royal Engineers, and was stationed in Germany after the Second World War, and in Malaysia.

My brother, Damian, has followed in the footsteps of our ancestors and has served in the parachute regiment for a number of years, going to Germany, Bosnia, Oman and, more recently, Afghanistan. So, for personal reasons, it meant a lot to me to have the opportunity to see the military in operation. It helped me understand a little more about the personalities in my family, and how important a role the men and women in the armed services have. It's imperative, too, that we remind people at home what's happening when the armed forces are posted abroad, whether it's in frontline service, or peace-keeping missions, and for that reason alone I was very proud and privileged to undertake a morale-boosting mission – it's also, of course, something that one of my heroines, Marilyn Monroe, had done before me.

The *Daily Star* flew us out under the banner 'Top Totty Tour of Bosnia', so Jo and I could act as Little Miss Christmas to the squaddies, handing out Christmas puddings, mince pies and crackers donated by Asda supermarket.

When we arrived in Sarajevo, we boarded a Chinook helicopter, piloted by two young British soldiers, who decided to show off with a load of crazy stunts as they flew us to visit the 1st Battalion King's Own Royal Border Regiment, who were working on the front line. Ironically, my brother was stationed out there at the time, as a seventeen-year-old soldier, not that he'd tell anyone I was his sister because all the men had our posters on their walls which made him feel a bit awkward to say the least. Thankfully I didn't see him during my visit: he wouldn't have known where to look if we had, considering I was saucily dressed as Mother Christmas!

left: Here I am at sweet sixteen, having just completed my GCSEs.

right: On an early calendar shoot; Alan Strutt and I have worked together for many years.

All the soldiers who were stationed in Bosnia were on a one-hour call-out, so even when they were off duty, there was always the potential that they could be called to action.

It was quite astounding to see the surrounding towns and villages, which had been bombed beyond recognition. I expected things to be bad, but seeing the reality was a real eye-opener for me and Jo. Lots of our land journeys were across minefields, so it was quite dangerous and really made us appreciate the perilous situations our servicemen and women face when they are on duty abroad.

Jo and I had quite a hectic schedule, with a whistle-stop tour of various bases, sleeping in barracks in the middle of winter when the temperatures were freezing, eating in the mess halls and having lots of fun, in spite of everything. We dressed up in sexy Santa outfits, with fishnet tights and fur-trimmed minidresses, then signed calendars and posed for pictures with the soldiers. In return for kisses and autographs, the troops put on shows for us, mimicking the Spice Girls and Village People and making us feel incredibly welcome.

It was a phenomenally emotional experience for me: I had just turned eighteen myself, and many of the soldiers we met were the same age as me. If we were able to bring a little cheer into their lives, I thought, that can only be a good thing.

The following Christmas, I got to repeat the experience, visiting HMS *Invincible*, which was stationed in the Mediterranean, off the coast of Cyprus. The *Sun* newspaper sent me out there to cheer up the Marines dressed as Mother Christmas once again.

Once my glamour modelling career took off, it was suggested I publish my own official Kelly Brook calendar, to build on my growing 'pin-up' status. I'd worked a lot with the photographer Alan Strutt, and he'd become a good friend as well as a professional colleague, so I asked if he'd be interested in working with me on the pictures. We've collaborated on various projects for over a decade now, and we still come up with new ideas and have a lot of fun working together, despite the challenges we often face when putting together a supposedly glamorous set of images for the official calendar, which we've produced since 2001.

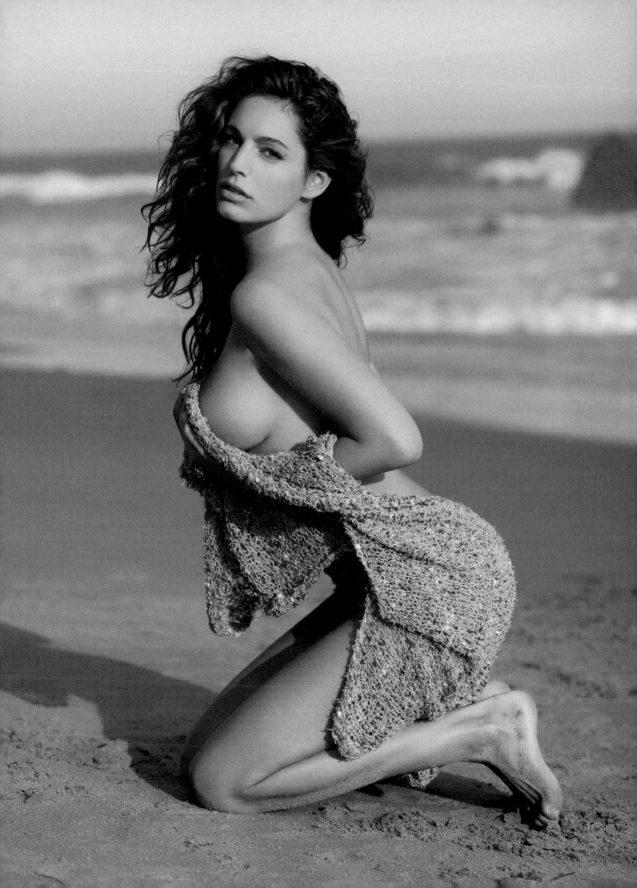

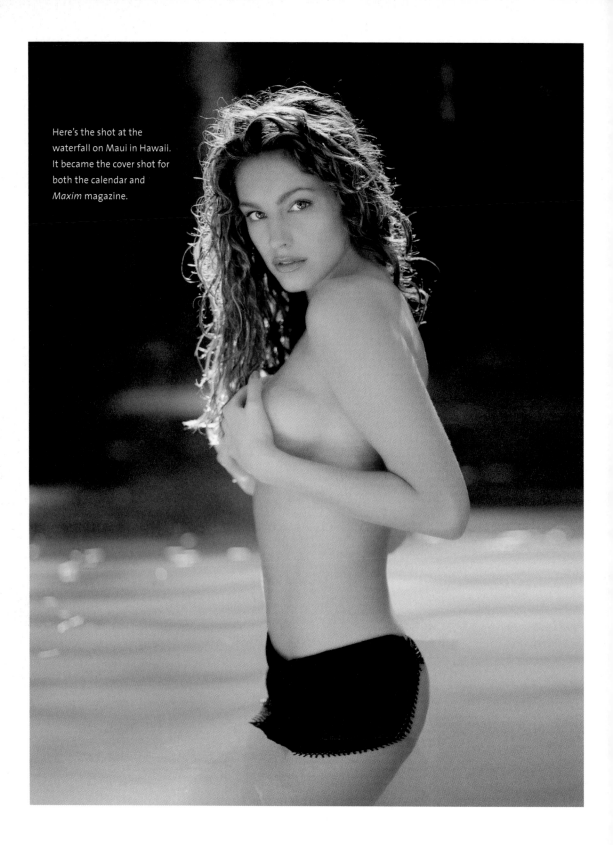

Here's the shot at the
waterfall on Maui in Hawaii.
It became the cover shot for
both the calendar and
Maxim magazine.

It can be quite an adventure producing the shots we need, as we're always on a tight budget and have to go somewhere exotic to get sunshine and beautiful locations. I don't always use a stylist for the calendars, as I have such a strong idea of the look I'm trying to achieve, so sometimes it's just easier to do it myself. Well, that's the idea, anyway.

One year, Alan and I decided to travel to Hawaii to shoot the calendar, as it wasn't too far from Hollywood, where I was living at the time, and we loved the idea of volcanic rock and waterfalls as a backdrop. After being there for a few days I was really unhappy with what we'd shot and was determined to find a waterfall so we could do the picture we'd envisaged. 'Why else come all this way?' I said to the team.

We were on the island of Maui at the time, and I asked the locals if they knew where we could find the perfect waterfall for our shot. Someone suggested a huge national park on the other side of the island, where they told us there was the most beautiful waterfall.

'Right,' I said, with renewed energy, trying to motivate everyone. 'Let's go.'

As we arrived at the park and enquired about the whereabouts of the waterfall, we discovered we had a hike ahead of us. The four of us – Alan and his assistant, with all their camera gear, Kim with her hair and make-up kit and me with my bags – trekked for what seemed like miles through swamps, over rocks and up hills. We were exhausted and extremely frustrated by the effort needed to reach this elusive waterfall.

When we eventually arrived, though, it was worth all the effort. The locals' descriptions of an idyllic waterfall were completely accurate: it was stunningly beautiful and a breathtaking sight.

As the day was getting on, we started to set up the equipment and get ready, but to my horror I discovered I'd bought the wrong bag, and the only thing in there of any use was a black neck scarf! Understandably, everyone looked like they wanted to kill me. Always the optimist, and feeling utterly sick with guilt, I confidently declared that I would resolve the situation. After all, it was a calendar shoot and I hadn't exactly planned to wear many clothes!

I wrapped the tiny piece of cloth around my waist, strategically positioned myself so I revealed nothing naughty, then perfected the 'hand bra', cupping my breasts in the palms of my hands. Alan, delighted finally to be taking pictures after our lengthy trek and the trauma of the non-existent bikinis, started snapping away. As the sun glistened in the tumbling waters, creating dancing rainbows amid the lush surroundings, we finally got the shot we wanted.

Just as everything was going perfectly, though, we heard noises in the distance. We looked up, and over the brow of the hill there appeared a Scout troop marching towards us. There were about thirty boys, probably only just in their teens, and as they got closer they proceeded to 'make camp' and settle down to their packed lunches overlooking our location. I'm sure it wasn't quite the view they'd anticipated, watching a near-naked girl frolicking in the water for a photographer, but they spent the rest of the day, until sundown in fact, watching us at work. I suspect their Hawaiian nature hike took on a whole new meaning that day!

One of the early jobs I got was with the computer games company Eidos. They flew me and some other actors and models out to Atlanta, Georgia, and New York, where we had to dress up as the characters from their games and act out various scenarios. Eidos were also launching a new game called Fighting Force, and for the media junket in Manhattan they flew in journalists from all over the world to witness the unveiling at a massive computer gaming convention.

As a PR stunt, myself and three other actors were briefed to 'hijack' the bus taking the journalists to the convention. The plan was for the bus to turn down a dark alley in Manhattan, where an actor posing as the 'baddie' would jump onboard and pretend to take the press hostage. Then three of us in computer game character costumes would save the day.

It was one of the most embarrassing jobs I've ever been booked to do, because the journalists – unsurprisingly – were terrified and totally bemused. They genuinely looked frightened for a while, as they had no idea what was going on. I don't know whether the scheme was deemed a success, but I wouldn't be surprised if it had backfired and all their goodwill from the media disappeared.

However, one good thing did come out of the experience – for me, at least. One of the people on the bus was a girl called Antonia Davies, who was the costume designer for the characters we were playing and the then girlfriend of *Big Breakfast* presenter Johnny Vaughan. We became friends, and kept in touch after the New York trip, and it was Antonia who I later discovered put my name forward as a potential co-host to present the show with Johnny when Denise Van Outen left in October 1998.

my big break

While I'd been really busy with modelling and promotional work, and was enjoying the rewards that came with it, I was still keen to pursue an acting career, as that's what I had always wanted to do. The little girl who wanted to go to stage school had grown up, but she still had dreams of performing, and they weren't going away.

I'd secured a job presenting a wacky youth show on cable TV, called *VPL* (Visible Panty Line), and on it I toured the UK, meeting quirky characters in the fashion industry. Among the more unusual moments was the time I had to talk to a stripper who made her costume out of an English breakfast, or the pubic wig maker I had to interview. It was very niche and not exactly high profile, so I was keen to find an agent who could help me build a proper career path.

One day, out of the blue, I received a phone call from Planet 24, the TV production company, co-owned by Bob Geldof, who made *The Big Breakfast*, asking me to go in and see them as they wanted me to audition for the role of co-host. There had been speculation in the press on a daily basis about who would step into Denise's shoes when she left – she and Johnny had great chemistry together, but Denise had tired of the early-morning alarm call and wanted to do something different. All sorts of big names were rumoured to be in the running, so I was surprised that the production company was asking to see me, a completely unknown teenage lingerie model.

part one: my life

49

Kelly Brook

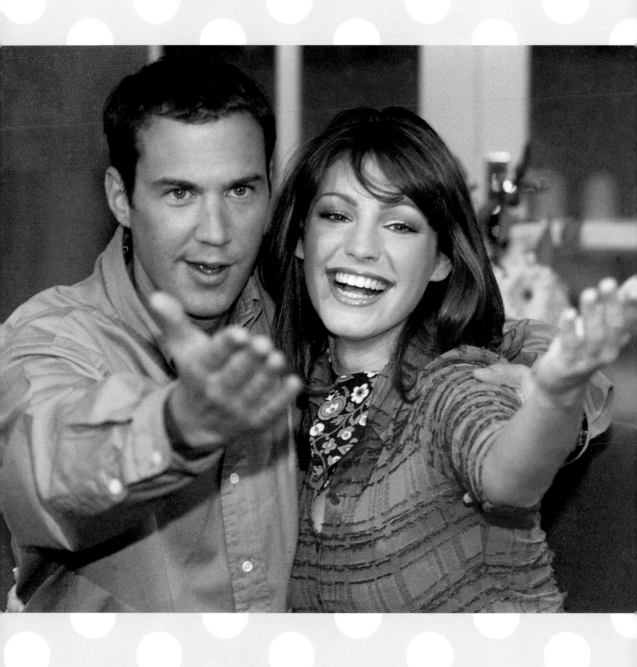

When I put the phone down, I stood there, shell-shocked. Surely they were fending off star names left, right and centre? It was only later I learned that Antonia had put my name forward.

When the time came to go along to Planet 24's head office and meet the producers, it was really intimidating, because *The Big Breakfast* was so well known. In its heyday, when Chris Evans and Gaby Roslin presented the show, they had daily audiences of about two million. The show itself was broadcast live from 7 a.m. to 9 a.m. five days a week from a set that was a former lock-keeper's cottage in east London. The show was renowned for its spontaneous, unscripted style, which required the team to think on their feet all the time.

Because of the press speculation about who was going to replace Denise – even the bookies were taking bets – I had to keep our meeting secret: Planet 24 sent a car to collect me and ushered me into the office via an underground car park. All the windows were blacked out in case there were paparazzi lurking, trying to see who was going in and out of their building. It all seemed rather silly to me at the time as I hadn't taken on board how important the job would be in terms of my career.

In our initial meeting, the producers asked me loads of questions and we chatted away about the kind of work I'd been doing and what I wanted to do with the rest of my life. I basically talked non-stop until they had to tell me to shut up, then, to my surprise, they asked me back to meet Johnny and do a screen test.

I returned to the studios a few days later and they put me in front of the cameras. During my screen test I managed to swear at least once and probably said all sorts of gossipy things that, had they been broadcast live on air, would have resulted in a flurry of libel suits. I was so excited I just couldn't dampen my enthusiasm, so I was convinced I'd completely messed up, and went home thinking it had just been good experience for the future. I took their 'we'll be in touch' line with the pinch of salt you expect at castings and auditions. Onwards and upwards, as they say!

When I received a call a few days later to tell me I would be the next female presenter of the show, I couldn't speak. I really couldn't believe it. I was standing in the kitchen at my parents' house – I was still living at home at that point – and my mum just turned to me and said, 'Oh my God, Kelly, you've never done live television, are you sure you can do this?'

What would you have done in my shoes? Would you think, I've never done much television work before, so don't bother, I might make a fool of myself? Or would you think, what a fantastic opportunity to see what I'm capable of. The producers think I can do it and I've got nothing to lose, so let's give it a go? It's a no-brainer really, isn't it?

left: A photocall with Johnny Vaughan when they announced me as his new co-host on *The Big Breakfast*.

Some people thought I'd bitten off more than I could chew, but the opportunity to co-present one of British television's hottest shows was too good to resist. It was also a regular job as opposed to intermittent modelling work, so it would provide me with a steady income and some independence.

On the day I signed my contract, I was invited to tea at the House of Lords with Waheed Ali, one of the founders of Planet 24, who'd been made a life peer a year earlier at the age of thirty-four. I couldn't believe my luck. I remember very clearly the day the news broke in the media. The front page of the *Sun* featured a huge picture of me in a black bra and knickers under the headline KELLYVISION.

Victoria Newton, a respected showbusiness journalist, had got the scoop on her rivals and was proud to declare her exclusive with the line 'Teenager is new Denise'. Inside, on page three, the paper compared me to Denise Van Outen, saying we both had 'a fabulous figure and the gift of the gab', and that I'd 'beaten' competition from TV babes Gail Porter, Melanie Sykes and Caprice to land the £200,000-a-year job.

right: The first issue of *Heat* magazine and our first interview together.

It was then that I got my first proper taste of celebrity as photographers camped outside my family home and our phone rang off the hook. My mum even made pots of tea for the photographers who'd camped outside our house since dawn to try to take my picture. I received countless bouquets of flowers and good luck cards, some from close friends and family, some from people I hadn't heard from in years, and others from complete strangers.

Before I went live on air for my first show on 1 February 1999, we did a series of run-throughs – 'as-live' shows that weren't actually broadcast – so I that could learn how the show worked. I had to familiarise myself with the different elements of the show and the layout of the house where it was filmed. As you can imagine, it wasn't as straightforward as working in an open TV studio.

THE ULTIMATE WEEKLY
ENTERTAINMENT FIX

NEW!

heat

£1.25 6-12 FEBRUARY 1999

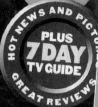

**SHAKESPEARE
IN LOVE**
The gags
you missed

SEX & THE CITY
Secrets of
episode five

GOLDEN GLOBES
Full report
& pictures

**SHARLEEN
SPITERI**
Soaking wet!

EXCLUSIVE
INTERVIEW &
PICTURES

WHEN KELLY
MET JOHNNY

Cooking up chemistry on *The Big Breakfast*

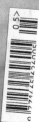

I also needed to get used to working while wearing an earpiece, which is how the director communicates with the presenters when they're live on air. It's quite off-putting when you're chatting away to the camera and the director is telling you something through your earpiece – I'd never appreciated that live TV presenters needed to be able to speak and listen to instructions at the same time, all the while looking as if they're behaving completely naturally. It was only then that it began to dawn on me what I'd let myself in for: this was a major job! And contrary to popular belief, there was no autocue.

The producers had asked if there was anything I wanted to do to make the show work better for me as a presenter, as everyone has a different style and preferences on how they like things to be done. I found that the scripts weren't written in the style in which I speak, and that it worked better when Johnny and I were left to chat unscripted, so I suggested they kept the scripts minimal, so we could banter on screen, and then I would rewrite the scripts each morning to suit my delivery, which is what most TV presenters do. That way, if there were words I don't use in day-to-day conversation, I could replace them with my own natural vocabulary.

right: My Triumph bra campaign: the tagline hinted at my new role on *The Big Breakfast*.

During my first week on the show, journalists were commissioned to sit and watch every second of output, breaking down and analysing every word and gesture I made, so they could critique my performance. I could almost feel the pressure as the cameras went live each morning, but with typical Kelly optimism, I kept reminding myself that it was a live show, and because I had no experience it would take a while to find my feet.

In the ensuing weeks as I got to grips with co-presenting the show, I came in for a fair bit of flack in the media. It might seem strange but I can honestly say I didn't let it get to me. One thing drama school really prepares you for is rejection, and I'd been drilled to expect criticism and had become pretty thick-skinned as a result. As far as I was concerned, I was learning on the job and enjoying all the perks that went with it: free clothes, a new car, interviewing amazing people and doing some really fun things. Some of the comments were hurtful, I'll admit, but I didn't sit crying in the corner, it just made me even more determined to learn the ropes and improve. After all, I'd never professed to be anything other than a young girl who'd been given an incredible chance to try a dream job. The only person I felt for during that time was Johnny, because there were a lot of comments in the media that the show wasn't

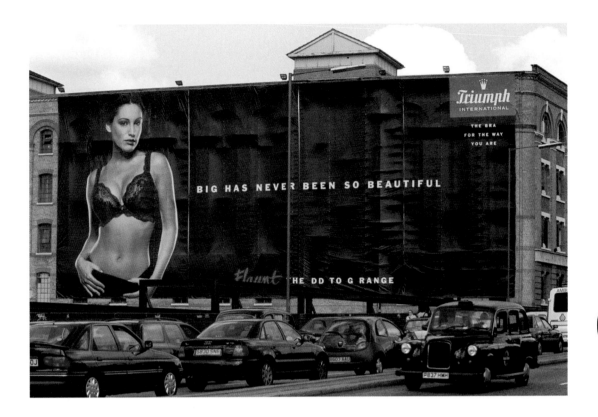

working now that Denise had left, which must have been hard for him.

When I first joined the *The Big Breakfast*, I wore a couple of outfits that were a bit risqué and there was a memo sent to the costume department suggesting I should cover up more. After that I started wearing below-the-knee skirts and covering my cleavage, which my friends and family thought was hilarious as I was a nineteen-year-old girl dressing like a mumsy librarian. My granny said to me, 'Why are you covering up your lovely figure?' and after I repeated this to Johnny, he made me tell the story on air. The memo also got leaked, and it started a national newspaper campaign to get me back into skimpy clothing. They agreed that it was ridiculous that the bosses wanted me to cover up. After all, I wasn't trying to be Kate Adie or anything, I was

supposed to be a bubbly young presenter on a fun, fast, fashionable breakfast show.

In the early days of *The Big Breakfast*, I was doing a lot of media work, so when I came off air at 9 a.m. I often went straight off to do photo shoots, interviews and other promotional work to plug the show, so that I didn't get home until about seven in the evening. Even my driver wasn't allowed to do the number of hours I was doing, so I would have to make my own way home in a cab to my mum and dad's house in Kent, totally exhausted.

It was really gruelling, and when I finally got home all I wanted to do was go to bed, but my parents wanted to know about my day and the phone would ring, so it was hard to get to sleep. In desperation I asked the cab company to tell the drivers not to talk to me because I needed to sleep on the journey home, and one of them said to me, 'I've been told not to talk to you', which made me sound like a real diva. As you can see, it's all too easy to be misinterpreted.

In spite of all this, though, I was having a fabulous time. To try to put me at ease, the production team had asked me to put together a list of my favourite people, so they could try to book them as guests on

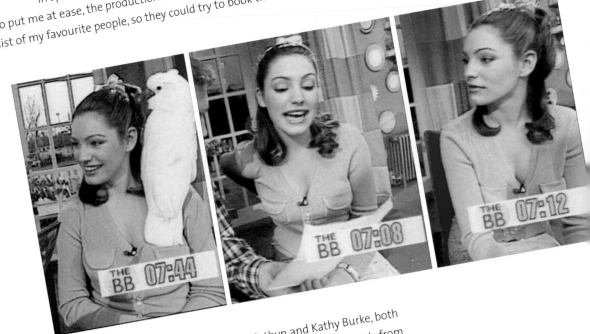

the show. My wish list included Brenda Blethyn and Kathy Burke, both amazing British actresses I'd long admired, and my schoolfriends from Italia Conti, Dannielle Brent (who's now a successful TV actress who starred in *Bad Girls*) and Natasha Green. All of them appeared on the show in my first week, which was very special for me as I tried to ease myself into my new role.

As time went on, I started to get into the spirit of the show and enjoy myself, and I interviewed a host of well-known names on the programme, from Hugh Grant and Ricky Martin to Salman Rushdie and Britney Spears. I had a wardrobe budget and a huge selection of bright and breezy breakfast television clothes, and the atmosphere on set was intense: there was often no knowing what was going to happen next. I remember one morning, I was in the middle of a live broadcast from *The Big Breakfast* garden – a regular feature when the weather was nice – when the producers in the gallery began screaming urgently in my

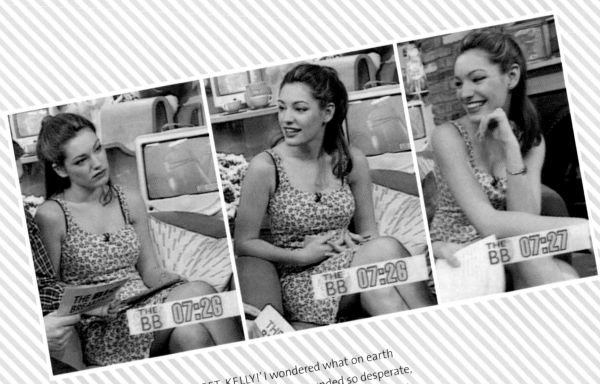

ear: 'Move left, Kelly! MOVE LEFT, KELLY!' I wondered what on earth was happening and couldn't work out why they sounded so desperate, until I noticed something out of the corner of my eye in the canal that ran alongside the garden. It later emerged that a dead body had been pulled from the water, but only after it had floated past me as we were on air. The joys of live television!

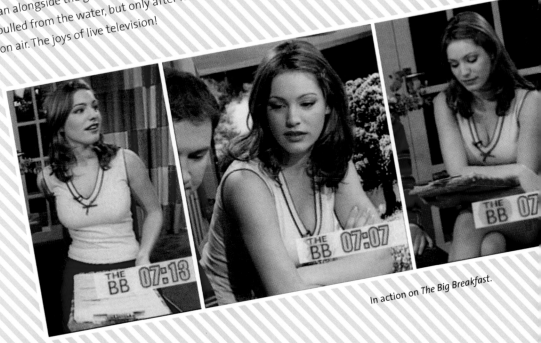

In action on *The Big Breakfast*.

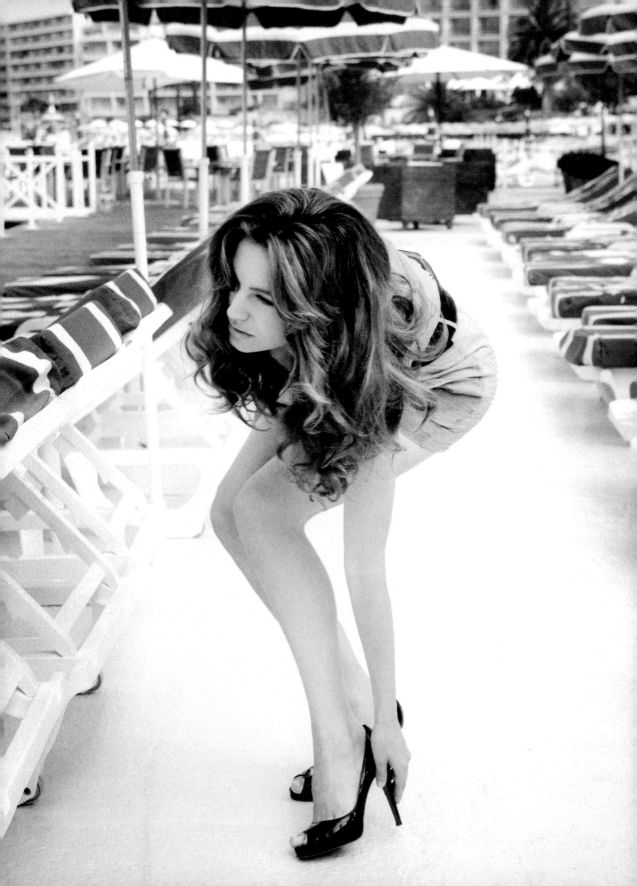

About six months after I joined *The Big Breakfast*, I took a much-needed fortnight's holiday with my then boyfriend, Jason Statham. I'd been working incredibly hard, getting up at 4 a.m. five days a week to do a live, adrenalin-fuelled show, and I was completely exhausted. We booked ourselves a sunshine break in Gran Canaria to visit Jason's parents, and I decided to try and forget about work: I was keen to relax completely, so I could start back refreshed and full of energy.

After a couple of days lazing by the pool and wandering along the beach with Jason, I finally started to switch off, forgetting all about life in London and my crazy early-morning alarm call. It was bliss. But my plans to leave reality behind while I enjoyed a romantic escape were about to be turned upside down.

On 28 July 1999, I went to the local shop to buy ice cream and saw a copy of the *Sun* out of the corner of my eye. I got the shock of my life. Splashed across the front page was the headline, 'ANOTHER SUN EXCLUSIVE – TV KELLY AXED – BIG BREKKIE GIRL GOES AFTER JUST SIX MONTHS'.

It was the first I knew of it and I was stunned. I went and sat on the beach with Jason and read the piece. Alongside a picture of me modelling Triumph lingerie, the text read, 'TV beauty Kelly Brook is to be sacked from her star role on *The Big Breakfast* after just six months, the *Sun* can reveal. The stunning 19-year-old is expected to be dropped as Johnny Vaughan's co-presenter when she comes back from a summer holiday.'

This was me they were writing about! It was incredibly surreal, but I sat, speechless, and read on. According to the article, I had been criticised since taking over from Denise Van Outen for various reasons. They quoted from a leaked memo that said I needed help with long words and tricky scripts, and I had apparently not developed the right on-screen chemistry with Johnny. It seemed that my replacements while I was on holiday had been instant successes with viewers. The paper claimed that I would be kept on in a minor role until the end of my contract.

Ironically, that early attempt to define my natural presenting style, and my request to keep scripts minimal so that Johnny and I could develop a relaxed, unscripted chemistry, had been completely distorted by the media after internal memos were leaked. I was horrified.

My confidence was completely crushed: although I knew there were times when we'd had hiccups on the show, we'd been having a lot of fun and the viewing figures were pretty stable. Johnny and I had become good mates – Jason and I were guests at his and Antonia's wedding the following month – and I'd been getting on well – or so I'd thought – with the production team and crew.

What's a girl to do? You're sitting poolside on your holiday, trying to catch a few rays with your boyfriend, when you read on the front page of the country's most popular newspaper that you're about to be sacked. I recalled the interview I'd done with the very same paper when I'd first got the *Big Breakfast* job: 'I'm well aware that some people have failed. It's all going to come down to whether people like me or not, and that's what's exciting. But if they don't like me, then at least I've had a go. Let's just hope I'm not crap.'

Clearly the story wasn't going to go away. Various options were open to me: I could ignore it and see what happened when we got back to England, but I was convinced the press would get to us on holiday before that, and then it wouldn't be a holiday any more; I could issue some kind of statement saying 'no comment'; or I could be dignified and walk away, holding my head up high.

I rang my mum and asked her advice. She didn't think I should go back and work at *The Big Breakfast*. She'd read the piece and felt it would be too much for me to go back as if nothing had happened. In the end I came to the conclusion that there would be other opportunities in the future; despite this one not having worked out, I knew what I was capable of, and would continue pursuing my dream. So, before Jason and I sat back and enjoyed the rest of our holiday, I took the bull by the horns and rang my bosses at Planet 24, handing in my resignation with immediate effect. I think they were a little shocked and even tried to tempt me back with an exclusive Will Smith interview – as if that was going to work.

Unfortunately, a few hiccups – especially when you're an attractive woman – is all the excuse the British need to knock you off the pedestal they've put you on, but I wasn't prepared to accept the limitations other people were trying to place on me. I would walk away from *The Big Breakfast* and prove my critics wrong. Although I'd suffered a blow, I would pick myself up, dust myself down and start all over again. Yes, my pride was hurt and my confidence took a blow, but I wasn't the first presenter to suffer a career setback, and I wouldn't be the last, either.

Before I came home from Spain, I bought a huge sombrero so the press wouldn't get the picture they wanted of me looking sad when I arrived back home from my holiday. Instead they got a ridiculous photo of me walking up the path at my mum and dad's house in a silly oversized Spanish hat.

After I'd left *The Big Breakfast*, I was offered the chance to answer my critics and write a piece, in my own words, in the *Mail on Sunday*, explaining how I felt about the furore. Here are some of the comments I made, under the headline:

why can't a woman have looks and a brain?

'I knew I had intelligence and the ability to achieve: I might not be an intellectual, but I have common sense and an enthusiasm for learning. I know the difference between an academic and someone who is smart: for example, my nan is clever. She could sit and talk to anyone about anything and has valid, informed opinions. She has a lifetime of experience to draw upon, but she can't quote a Hamlet soliloquy. And it would be an intellectual snob who suggested that made her stupid.

'I am nineteen years old, and have not attended life's college for very long. I do not profess to have an encyclopaedic knowledge of an array of subjects and there are words I struggle to pronounce. But I am fairly streetwise and have the kind of life experiences and interests that much of our audience might have related to.

'The thing is – and this is something that really annoys me – a lot of people mistake lightness for stupidity. If you're cold and mean and dark, you're smart. If you're sweet and charming and you get on with people, then you're not. Then, you're described as bubbly and thick.

'I also believe class and accent were another factor in my downfall: my Estuary vowels gave the critics as many slings and arrows as my supposed ignorance. But Queen's English is no more an indication of intellect than a pair of geeky spectacles: there are plenty of well-spoken idiots out there, while the likes of Ben Elton and Kathy Burke hardly speak with received pronunciation but are rightly credited with being gifted and bright.'

Once I'd returned from my holiday, I decided to try to get myself on the books of an acting agency. My childhood dream had always been to act, and it was something I still hankered after. The William Morris Agency, which is one of the best-known showbusiness agencies in the world, with offices in London, New York, Beverly Hills, Nashville, Miami Beach and Shanghai, took me on, and the woman assigned to me said they would look out for appropriate television and film roles – perhaps even theatre – but wanted me to sign with their presenters' division, too. She felt that people no longer got pigeon-holed as a 'presenter' or an 'actor', and that if I could raise my profile in either sphere it would help me get where I wanted to be.

right: A publicity shot for my MTV show, *Select*.

Initially I was reluctant to consider presenting jobs at all. *The Big Breakfast* had been great fun but it had turned sour so quickly and left a bitter taste in my mouth. I wasn't ready to put myself in line for ridicule again. However, I had to take my agents' advice: they were the experts after all, so I signed up and they told me MTV were looking for a VJ to host her own show. I was understandably cautious, but my new agent sat me down and said firmly, 'Kelly, it's like riding a bike. You fall off, but you have to get straight back on again.'

In the end I was persuaded to give it a go, and went along to the MTV studios in Camden, north London, to try out for the job. The next thing I knew, I was hosting my own show called *Select*, a two-hour live programme where I got to interview fab people and play great music.

Like *The Big Breakfast*, it was a youth-orientated, fast-paced show, but I felt more at home there, and somehow it went more smoothly. I'd learned a lot from my six months' experience with Planet 24, but it was presenting my own show at MTV that gave my confidence the boost it needed, and after eighteen months there, I finally felt that the world was at my feet.

'you fall off, bu
to get straight

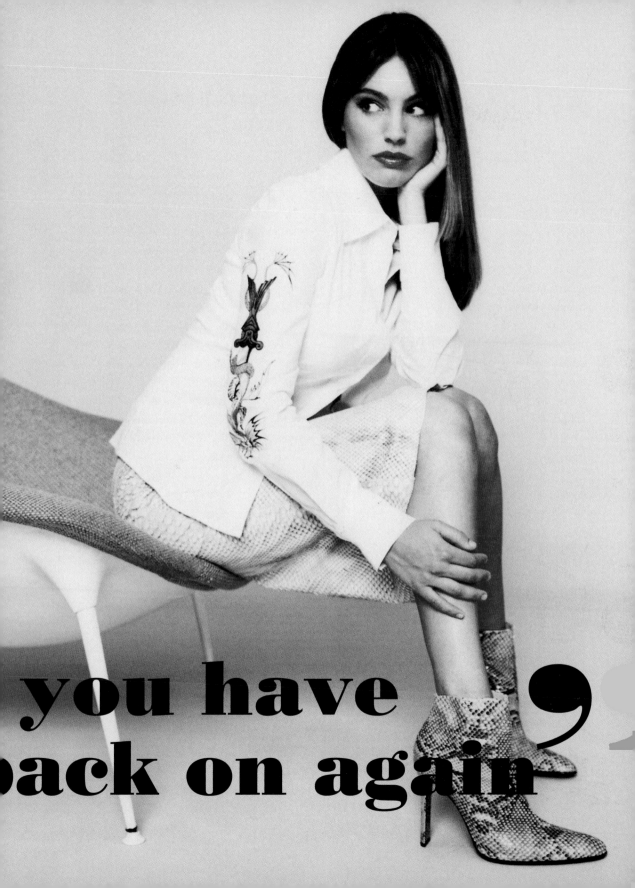

you have
back on again

getting sorted for hollywood

below: The programme
for *Eye Contact*.

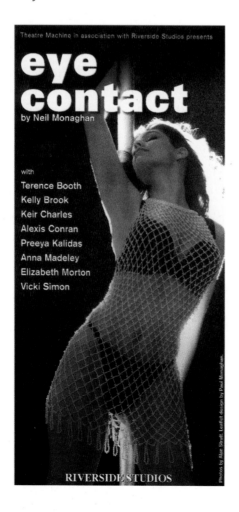

Theatre Machine in association with Riverside Studios presents

eye contact
by Neil Monaghan

with
Terence Booth
Kelly Brook
Keir Charles
Alexis Conran
Preeya Kalidas
Anna Madeley
Elizabeth Morton
Vicki Simon

RIVERSIDE STUDIOS

Photos by Alan Strutt. Leaflet design by Paul Monaghan.

During my time at MTV, I continued to audition for various roles that William Morris put me up for as I was still determined to pursue my goal to act. I made my feature film debut in 2000, in a British-made thriller called *Sorted*, which was the story of a young lawyer, played by Matthew Rhys, investigating his brother's untimely death. I played the small part of Sarah, acting alongside Sienna Guillory and Jason Donovan, which gave me my entrée into the world of the big screen.

I also auditioned for a stage play, *Eye Contact*, which was a drama about the sexual politics at a table-dancing club and the unfolding relationships between the punters and the club's dancers. Written by Neil Monaghan, a highly regarded young scriptwriter, it was a controversial contemporary play, and I was thrilled when I won the part of a lap dancer called Anya.

I had to learn to pole dance, so I went for lessons with some of the professional dancers at the Astral Club in London's Soho. I remember realising very quickly that it was much harder than it looked and that these girls were extremely talented performers. Rehearsals soon got started, and I would come home black and blue from contorting my body into different positions; it was exhausting.

The play was scheduled for a run at the Riverside Theatre in Hammersmith, west London: it's quite a serious arts theatre and I think we raised a few eyebrows among their regulars by putting on a play about strippers. Our opening night was 23 November 2000, which was my twenty-first birthday – little did I imagine I'd be celebrating this landmark birthday by cavorting semi-naked around a pole, in front of an audience of theatre critics.

Playing the lead
role in the rather risqué
performance, *Eye Contact*.

The production received mixed reviews,
and on a personal level a lot of critics seemed to have
formed an opinion about me well before they took
their seats to watch the play, while others clearly
came with an open mind and offered a fair assess-
ment. The cast and crew, however, were delighted
when the show sold out for its initial run and we
had to extend the dates.

It was obvious that some people came just
to be voyeurs, but if that was what it took to get
teenage boys out of bars and pubs to sample a little
culture, that's no bad thing. However, I was conscious
of the disappointment when I finished my dance on
stage each night: you could hear a ripple of voices
asking, 'Is that it...?' Some of the audience obviously
expected to see more than they did – I bared my top
half, but didn't get fully starkers – and I sometimes
felt as if I'd let them down.

One day while making *Sorted*, I found myself
sitting next to Tim Curry at lunch. Best known for his
role as Frank-N-Furter in *The Rocky Horror Picture
Show*, he started to tell me about his life in
Hollywood, saying that if I were ever to find myself
there I should give his manager, Joan Hyler, a call.
By coincidence, Jason had been invited out to Los
Angeles to meet some studio executives after the
success of Guy Ritchie's movie, *Lock, Stock and Two
Smoking Barrels*, and it seemed like a fantastic
opportunity for us both. I'd been at MTV for nearly
eighteen months and was desperate for a change,
so I handed in my resignation and bought a plane
ticket to Los Angeles.

We stayed in a guest house in Malibu and I drove all over LA, accompanying Jason to his meetings, and eventually I decided to pull out Joan's number and arrange to meet up with her. On our first meeting I was really honest and told her about my trip from beauty queen to TV host, adding that I was really keen to spend some time in LA after I'd fulfilled my contract with MTV and the play I'd signed up to appear in.

Back home, as my final appearances in *Eye Contact* loomed, I heard via Joan that there was an opportunity for a television role in the US. It was a pilot for a show called *The (Mis)Adventures of Fiona Plum*, and they had just lost their original leading lady. It was a sitcom about a British witch who'd been sent to America to work as a nanny for three children – *Mary Poppins* meets *Bewitched* meets *I Love Lucy*. I had to have that role! I'd always loved Lucille Ball in *I Love Lucy*, and I used to dream of creating a persona like that: it was the perfect opportunity.

I'd never done any comedy before, and the idea of doing an American TV show was somewhat different to working on the London stage or presenting on MTV, but I was completely deter-mined to make the role of Fiona Plum mine, and did everything I could to give myself the best chance of landing the job. First I booked a plane ticket to Los Angeles, then I spent three weeks creating the character I believed would work for Fiona Plum, perfecting her voice, her nuances and her expressions. I lived, breathed, slept, shopped and ate as Fiona Plum – in short, I became her.

In America, the casting process is a huge deal and it's incredibly intimidating. First you meet and audition with the casting director, then, if you make the grade, you meet and audition with the producers. If they like you, they send you along to meet the studio bosses. And then, if you're still in the running, you audition for the TV network bosses – after all, they hold the purse strings, and they know their audiences.

The whole process is seriously hard work and very draining, but each time you get to the next stage, there's an overwhelming sense of excitement. I so desperately wanted the job that I was filled with fear every time I went to a meeting and couldn't contain my joy each time I got to the next tier of the process.

Eventually, I'd climbed every nerve-racking rung of the casting ladder and seen everyone that needed to be seen in order to get the part, which meant I just had to wait for that call. It was agony. Every time my mobile rang, I jumped out of my skin, wondering if this was going to be the all-important news.

Then, three weeks after I arrived in Hollywood, I got the call to tell me I had landed my first role. I was to play Fiona Plum. Kelly Brook, the glamour girl who'd become a laughing stock in London after *The Big Breakfast*, had just secured her own sitcom on network TV in America.

right: I was delighted that my acting career got off to such an encouraging start.

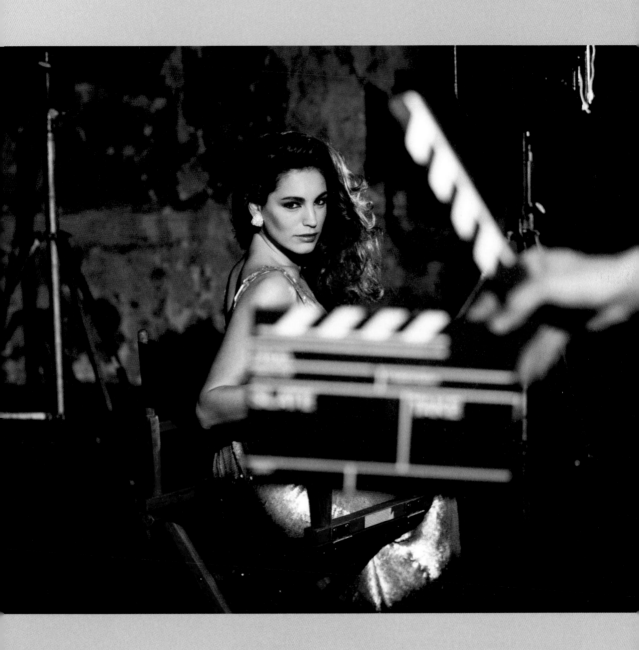

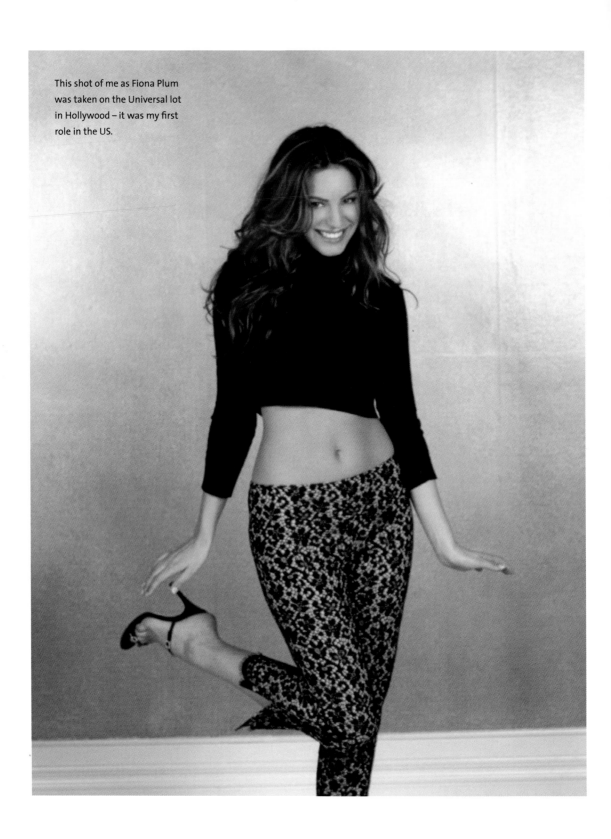

This shot of me as Fiona Plum was taken on the Universal lot in Hollywood – it was my first role in the US.

Inevitably, the British press went crazy; suddenly they wanted to know me again. I was no longer a failed breakfast TV presenter who couldn't string two words together, I was the latest starlet to make it big Stateside. How fickle, I thought to myself. So when I received a request from *The Big Breakfast* to be interviewed as a guest on their final show, I simply sent a memo saying, 'Sorry – gone to Hollywood!' You can imagine the pleasure that gave me.

One of the exciting things about taking on a new role is the opportunity to create a visual identity for the character, as well as working on elements of their personality. Once I'd secured the role of Fiona Plum, which was largely inspired by my love of Lucille Ball, I worked with the costume designer Bambi Breakstone – who was responsible for Don Johnson's wardrobe in *Miami Vice* back in the Eighties, though I never held that against her – to come up with a wardrobe that reflected the slightly kitsch retro mood I felt Fiona needed.

It was during this time that I paid my first visit to a vast vintage emporium on La Brea Avenue in Los Angeles. Bambi and I went together to try on lots of different styles and work on a look for Fiona Plum, and as we created 'yes' and 'no' piles, we rapidly realised that everything we liked was from the Fifties. We rummaged through racks and racks of amazing clothing, and it was then that I realised how much the 1950s silhouette, with its defined hourglass shape, suits my figure. We went on to replicate many of the pieces we found in contemporary fabrics, and ever since I've used the Fifties as a starting point for many of my looks, whether it's daywear, evening, beach or lingerie.

We shot the *Fiona Plum* pilot, with Michael York as my father, in the Universal lot, probably the most famous movie studio facilities in Hollywood. I was like a little girl at Christmas as I arrived for my first day on set, and the Universal lot was exactly as I'd imagined it, with big security gates, vast sound stages, personal parking places for the directors, and streets – it really is a small village – named after famous Hollywood stars.

The TV network had commissioned a full season of shows, and we were all ready to shoot when, out of the blue, the head of the network left. After that, to my great disappointment, they decided not to go ahead and shoot the series, so I never got to make *Fiona Plum* a reality beyond the pilot. It was such a shame, but at least I got paid for the full season, thanks to my new manager, Joan Hyler, and it had given me a taste for Hollywood and the opportunities that lay ahead.

When the network scrapped *Fiona Plum*, they cheered me up with some good news: they had another part for me. The series was called *Smallville*, and was based on the life of a young Clark Kent and his alter ego, Superman, who's coming to terms with who he is as a teenager. Tom Welling was Clark Kent and I was cast as Victoria Hardwick, the girlfriend of Lex Luthor, played by Michael Rosenbaum, and my brief was to be the ultimate femme fatale.

right: In action while making *Smallville*.
below: Here I am in Vancouver on the set of *Smallville* with Tom Welling and Michael Rosenbaum.

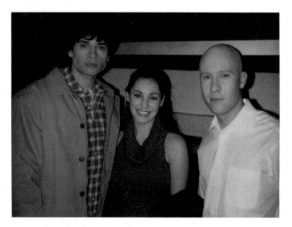

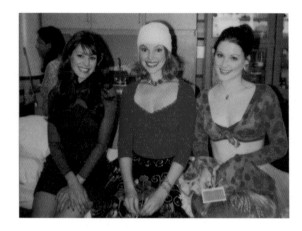

above: In *Romy and Michelle* with Katherine Heigl. Our outfits were all authentic Eighties pieces.

We shot on location in Vancouver, Canada, and I featured in four episodes, which appeared in 2002, with *Rolling Stone* magazine describing my character's impact as 'the best episodes of Lex Luthor's life'. The series was really popular, running for 133 episodes and winning two Emmy awards, the television equivalent of the Oscars. It also featured guest stars from the original *Superman* movies, such as Terence Stamp, Margot Kidder and even Christopher Reeve as a character called Dr Virgil Swann.

After *Smallville* my acting career really began to take off and I was regularly asked to attend castings and auditions for film and TV roles instead of having to beg to be seen. Finally, I was on the radar of some influential casting agents and directors. I travelled the world and visited some amazing places, including Mexico, France, Italy, Canada and even Romania. With Jason's career also blossoming, it was often difficult for us to see as much of each other as we would have liked.

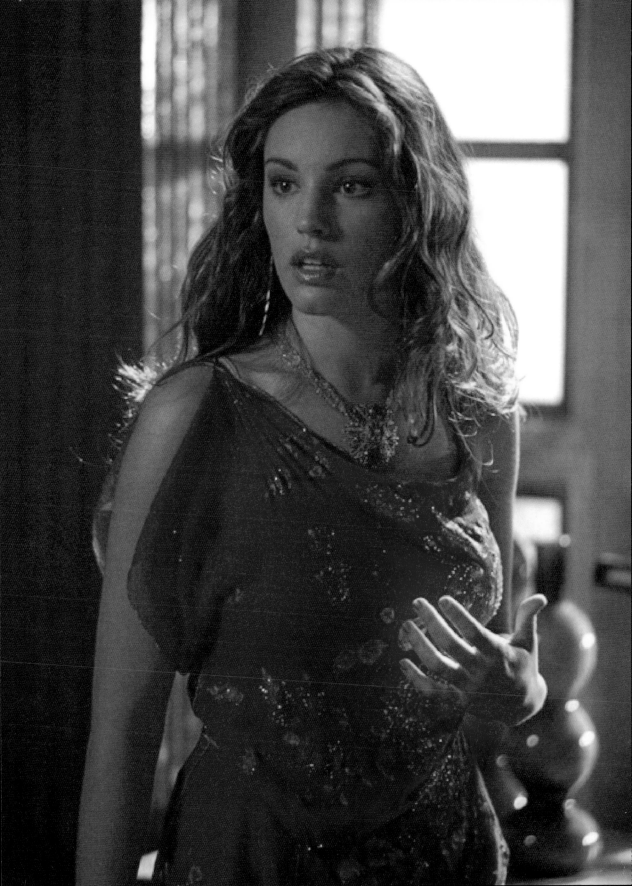

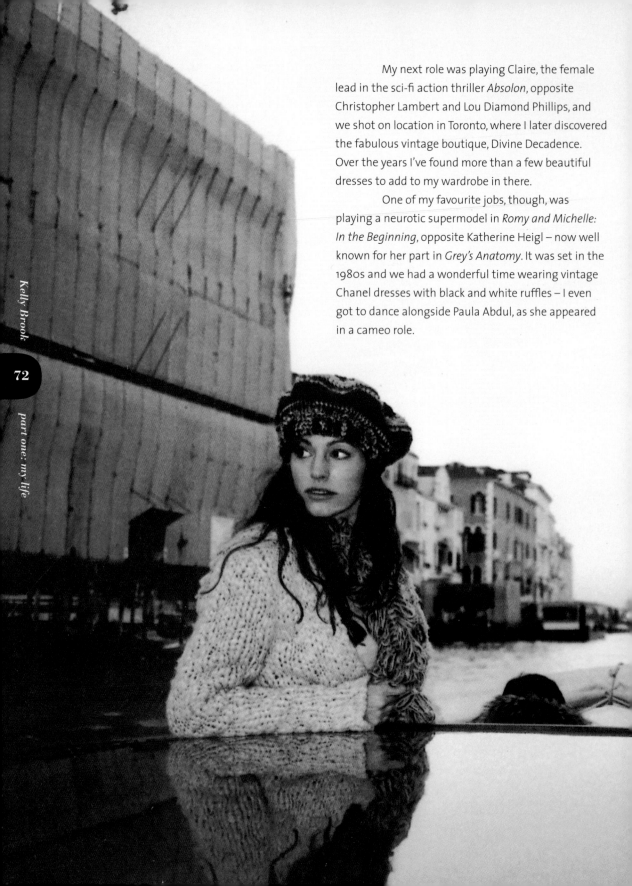

My next role was playing Claire, the female
lead in the sci-fi action thriller *Absolon*, opposite
Christopher Lambert and Lou Diamond Phillips, and
we shot on location in Toronto, where I later discovered
the fabulous vintage boutique, Divine Decadence.
Over the years I've found more than a few beautiful
dresses to add to my wardrobe in there.

One of my favourite jobs, though, was
playing a neurotic supermodel in *Romy and Michelle:
In the Beginning*, opposite Katherine Heigl – now well
known for her part in *Grey's Anatomy*. It was set in the
1980s and we had a wonderful time wearing vintage
Chanel dresses with black and white ruffles – I even
got to dance alongside Paula Abdul, as she appeared
in a cameo role.

In 2003 I was on holiday in Fiji – have you noticed how everything major in my career seems to happen while I'm on vacation? – when a complete film script came through on the hotel fax, addressed to me. The British writer/director Sue Heel wanted me for the lead role in her new movie *School for Seduction*, but she needed an answer right away, so I sat down and started reading immediately. I completely fell in love with the story about an Italian temptress called Sophia, who arrives in Newcastle-upon-Tyne to teach a group of Geordies the art of romance.

School for Seduction ticked all the boxes for me: it was charming, funny and celebrated womanhood in all its forms. It deals with issues such as being confident in who you are and at ease with your sexuality, no matter whether you're rich or poor, black or white, and I loved that idea. Not only that, I got to play a sultry Italian goddess called Sophia. That sealed the deal for me!

Sophia Loren has always been my favourite actress, so I called my agent immediately and said yes to the part. I simply *had* to do it. The only problem was I was English, with a very definite Estuary accent, while the part called for an Italian accent.

this page: In Venice, visiting Jason on set during the remake of *The Italian Job*.

inset: Filming *The Italian Job* on the Paramount lot in Hollywood, with Jason and Second Unit Director Alexander Witt.

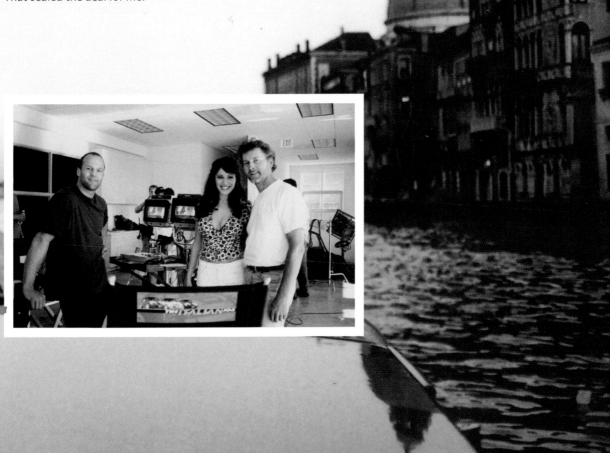

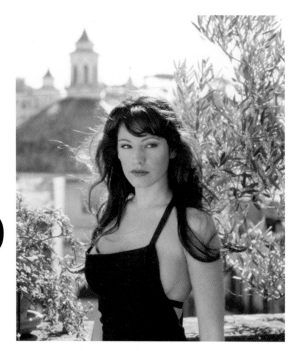

Above and opposite: As Sophia
on location in Rome in *School for
Seduction*; a scene from the
same film.

When I returned to LA after my holiday, I
worked with Michael Buster, a very well-known and
respected dialect coach, who introduced me to the
work of Italian actress Anna Magnani – I became a
big fan of her film *The Rose Tattoo*. I also studied all
of Sophia Loren's movies again to perfect my accent,
which reminded me how much I loved her deeply
sensual screen presence, especially in the 1960 classic
La Ciociara, known in the UK and US as *Two Women*,
for which she won an Oscar.

As well as practising my accent, I changed
my look to suit my Italian character. Daniel Galvin
Junior, who has been colouring my hair for years,
transformed my post-holiday sun-kissed golden locks
into a deep auburn, Mediterranean mane, and we
decided to cut a fringe in too.

The costume designer, Sally Plum, took me
to Céline, where Michael Kors was the chief designer,
and found a really gorgeous capsule wardrobe that
worked perfectly for the part. It was very glamorous
and sophisticated, and I loved the fact that it was a
classic elegant look. It really stood the test of time,
too, unlike my trendy wardrobe on MTV, which was
totally disposable.

The film was great fun: the cast included
Dervla Kirwan, Margi Clarke, Emily Woof and Tim
Healy, and we shot on location in Rome and the
north-east of England – you couldn't have had two
bigger contrasts! I loved shooting in Rome, wearing
glamorous clothes in the sunshine and eating
wonderful Italian ice cream. It was a heavenly movie
experience for me and my perfect acting role. Rome
is definitely one of my favourite cities in the world:
I love the architecture, the food and the chic lifestyle
of the people who live there, and it's incredibly
romantic.

After completing *School for Seduction*, my agent Andrew Ruff suggested I fly to Los Angeles for another pilot season. He told me a client of his, Billy Zane, was attached to a film being shot in the Bahamas, and was looking for a female lead. Andrew arranged a meeting for the afternoon of 24 February 2004 at the Chateau Marmont in Beverly Hills, which turned out to be Billy's thirty-eighth birthday.

Billy arrived fifteen minutes late, which I now know is impressive, given his dreadful time-keeping. He spotted me, smiled, then fell over as he walked down the stairs towards me. It was an interesting start to a meeting between strangers. We ordered afternoon tea and spoke at length about the script for *Three*, which was a sexy psychological thriller about a millionaire, Jack, played by Billy, and his wife Jennifer, which was the part I was reading, who are on a luxury yacht which ends up shipwrecked after an accident at sea. When we eventually parted later that afternoon, I left feeling I wasn't quite ready for this role, but I'm always open-minded and believe things happen for a reason, so I vowed to wait and see what happened.

The next day, I received a call saying that the director Stewart Raffill wanted to see me and put me on tape. I flew to London, did an audition with Juan Pablo Di Pace, who was playing the third lead, and within I week I had the part.

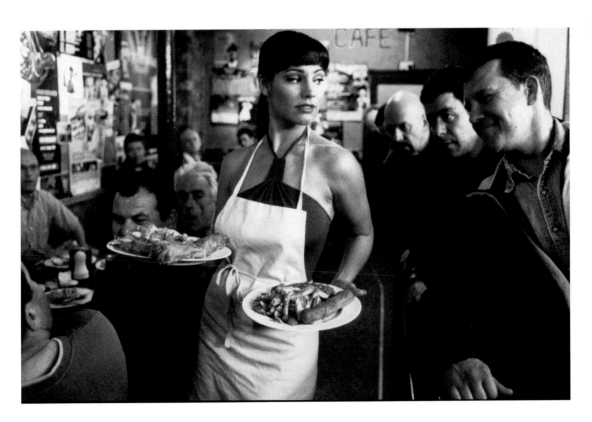

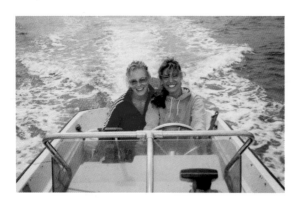

Once again I needed to work with a voice coach, because I was playing an American and needed to perfect the accent. I also had to prepare myself physically for the role, and booked in for a stint at Barry's Bootcamp in LA to get myself in shape before we flew to Eleuthera in the Bahamas on Easter Sunday. Barry's Bootcamp is an intense, get-yourself-in-shape, military-style programme many actors use when they need to get their bodies camera-ready, especially if they're short on time. Fans include Katie Holmes, Teri Hatcher, Jake Gyllenhaal, Alicia Silverstone, Jamie Lee Curtis, Hugh Jackman, Greg Kinnear and Nicollette Sheridan, who've all checked in to tone, slim and strengthen their bodies.

I took my friend Sadie with me to the Bahamas to keep me company while we were filming, and we couldn't have been in a more beautiful location. The beaches were long stretches of pale pink sand, and the water was a deep azure blue: it's easy to see why stars like Elle Macpherson, Christie Brinkley, Michelle Pfeiffer and the fashion designer Diane von Furstenberg are regular visitors to this island paradise off the coast of Florida.

While I was in the Bahamas, Jason was again filming on location elsewhere, and like so many other couples, it became clear that our relationship was faltering at the hands of the Hollywood lifestyle. We'd spent long periods apart due to work commitments, and when I returned to England for a fortnight, after seven years together we decided to call it a day.

When *Three* was released – it was called *Survival Island* in the UK – there were huge promotional posters plastered across the country, featuring a life-sized photo of me in a bikini, and it soon became apparent they were hot property, as they were taken down as fast as they were put up! There was even CCTV footage posted on the internet of a hoodie walking brazenly out of a shopping mall, with 'me' under his arm!

Soon after completing *Three*, I had a meeting with Adam Sandler's production company Happy Madison and won a part in *Deuce Bigalow: European Gigolo*, which we filmed in Amsterdam. But this was going to be my last film role for a little while as I was about to return to presenting a TV show.

above: My friend Sadie and me in the Bahamas, during downtime while filming *Three*.

right: The *Three* poster really was life-sized!

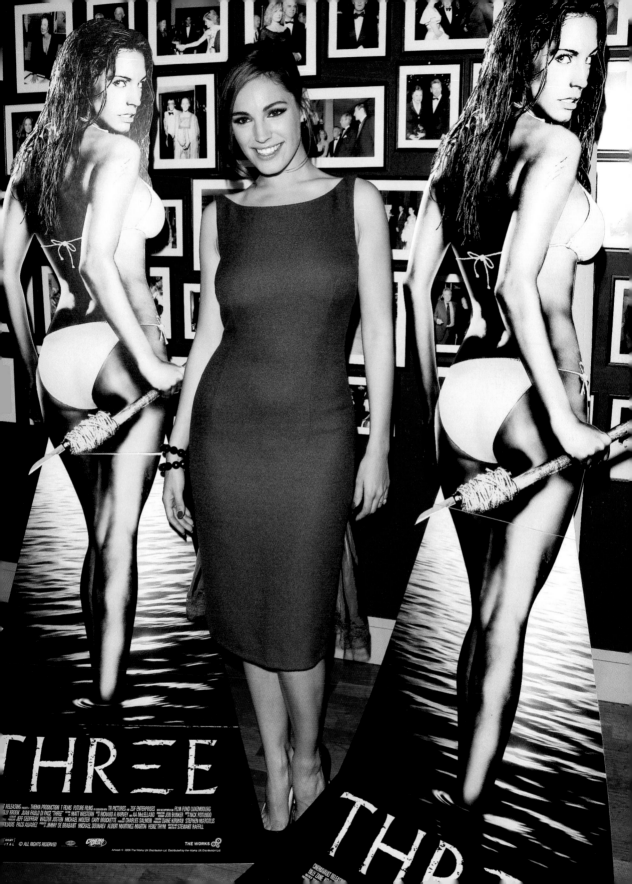

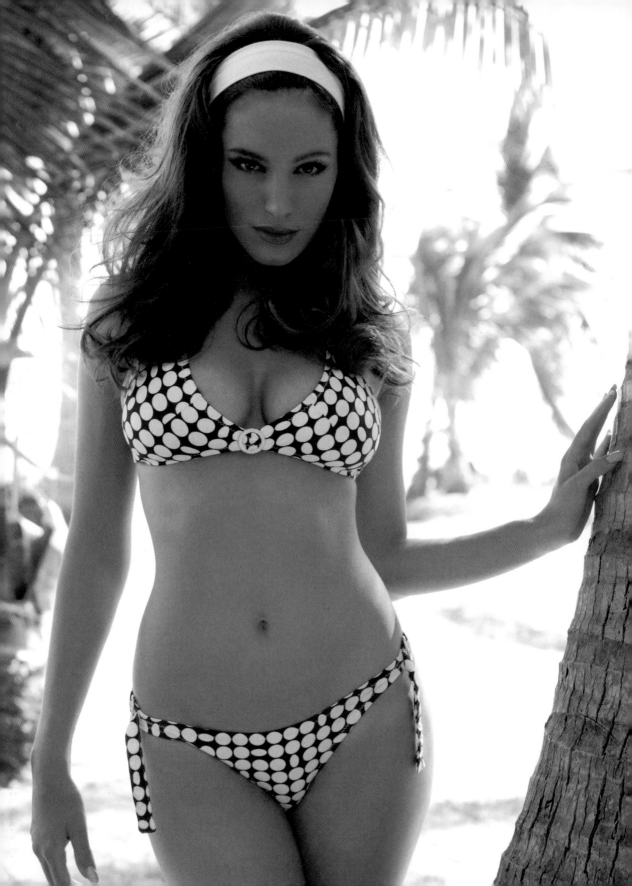

celebrity love island

07

What had happened was that while I was doing the rounds of castings and meetings for the Los Angeles pilot season in February 2005, my UK agent rang to tell me there was a new ITV reality show about to be commissioned called *Celebrity Love Island*, and asked if I'd be interested in co-presenting it?

At the time I was getting a fairly steady flow of acting jobs and hadn't given the idea of presenting a second thought as I was keen to try out for more American TV shows and establish myself properly as an actress in the US. But then the *Love Island* producer, Natalka Znak, flew out to meet me in Hollywood, and when she told me the location for the programme would be Fiji, I confess I was tempted. I'd been there before on holiday, and fell in love with it, so the opportunity to go again was too good to resist.

After a lot of thought, I decided I had nothing to lose, so I agreed and signed the contract. I spent a short time in London before we left for the South Pacific, and it was then that I met my co-host Patrick Kielty for the first time. The producers held a lunch for us, so we could get to know each other on 'home territory' before setting off for the remote island location that would be our base for the coming weeks.

I also asked the stylist Marcella Martinelli to help me with my wardrobe for the programme – I'd been given a clothing allowance, and was determined to have fun playing with different styles and creating a look for the show. We trawled vintage clothing shops and pulled together ideas from my favourite pin-ups, trying to combine the glamour of Raquel Welch in the Seventies – all big hair and smoky eyes – with early Bond girls like Claudine Auger, who starred opposite Sean Connery in *Thunderball*.

I then threw into the mix some of my favourite photos of Rita Hayworth, taken in the South Pacific in the Fifties. We wanted a sexy but wholesome look that was glamorous and appropriate for our location, so we took lots of vintage ruched 1950s swimsuits and tropical floral prints with us. I can't tell you how much fun we had putting together each day's outfit.

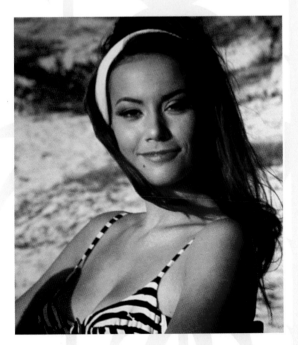

left: Claudine Augur as Dominique Derval in *Thunderball*. And me in a bikini inspired by her look.

When we returned to LA soon after filming *Love Island*, I rented a movie called *Son of Fury* and was amazed at how I'd managed to replicate most of the looks in that film – even down to the stripy shirts Billy wore most days – without ever having seen it.

By this time, Billy and I had developed a relationship and I was thrilled he had decided to come with me to Fiji: he said the opportunity to hang out in a tropical paradise watching me work was pretty hard to resist. Knowing I could be with him when I was off duty made the prospect of the weeks ahead even more exciting.

The set for *Love Island* was built on a small, private Fijian island, and the crew was staying on the main island, so we had to take a boat into work every day at 4 a.m. so that we were ready to go live at 8 p.m. UK time. It was very odd going back to my *Big Breakfast* hours, with the alarm going off at 3.30 a.m., and I'd really have to motivate myself to get out of bed as it was the last thing I felt like doing. If I'm honest, though, the idea of taking a boat out on the Pacific and spending the day on an idyllic beach fringed with palm trees was rather more appealing than a taxi drive through London and a morning on an East End canal!

this page and opposite: The movie *Mutiny on the Bounty* heavily influenced my wardrobe for *Celebrity Love Island*.

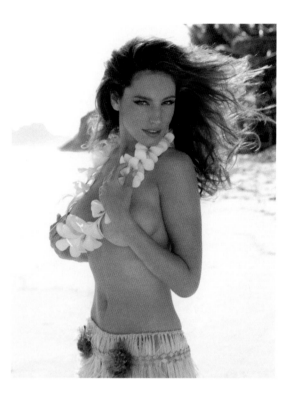
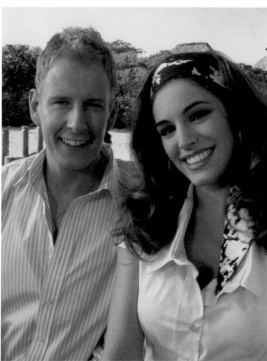

Before we went live with the show, we had a couple of weeks' rehearsals, which was useful in terms of developing on-screen chemistry with Patrick. He had vast experience hosting live television shows, while I hadn't done any for a few years and needed a little coaxing back into it. Patrick is fantastic to work with, and if the autocue were to break down or some other mishap were to happen while we were live on air, there's no one else I'd rather be sitting next to. We developed a friendship and trust that made the work feel like second nature, and we both really enjoyed the experience of filming *Love Island*, even though I was often the brunt of his jokes!

Once the show went live, our days settled into a routine: we'd all be on the boat at 4 a.m., but we were finished work by 9.30 a.m. so that the day was ours to do as we pleased. What a dream job! Billy and I would go off exploring, hanging out with the locals and visiting the tiny schools that nestled in the coastline of the islands. We chartered a helicopter and visited other islands like Turtle Island, which was used as the location for the Brooke Shields movie *Blue Lagoon* – and yes, it really was like the film.

above: With Patrick Kielty for *Celebrity Love Island.*

On one of our excursions, we discovered a beautiful island called Matamanoa, which I decided would be a stunning location for my 2006 calendar, so I rang Danilo, who produces the calendar, and organised for the photographic team to join us in Fiji. So, one day, after filming for *Love Island* had finished for the day, we took a boat across to Matamanoa, which was a forty-five-minute journey, and spent the day shooting pictures for the calendar. The weather was beautiful and we found plenty of stunning backdrops so that everyone was thrilled with the results of our day's work.

Late in the afternoon, our captain suggested we think about leaving as a storm was brewing, so we gathered our kit together and set off back to our island. Only fifteen minutes into the journey, the water started to get a little choppy, so the boat had to slow down, and forty-five minutes later we were getting nowhere fast. Then rain like I've never seen before started to fall. It was torrential, the sort of thing you see only in films. Before long we were in a severe storm and miles from anywhere.

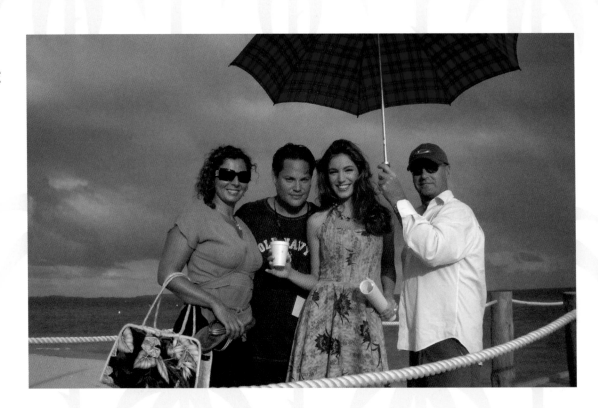

We all put our life jackets on, and Billy took it upon himself to be authoritative and try to keep everyone calm, but as we'd all seen him in *Dead Calm* and *Titanic*, it seemed strangely ironic for him to be giving us a speech about how we were perfectly safe!

At one point I heard someone scream, 'Oh my God! We're going down!' as we clung to each other for dear life. It felt like the boat was surfing enormous waves, and we were all pretty frightened. By this time, we'd been on board for over two hours and were desperate to get back on dry land. When we eventually did get back to base, we were soaked through and physically exhausted. Given his film roles, everyone else blamed Billy for bringing us bad luck and vowed never to set foot on a boat with him again – not an option that is open to me.

below left: The glam squad: in Fiji with stylist Marcella Martinelli, make-up artist Kim Goodwin and hairdresser Jonathon Malone.

below: This photo was taken at 6.30 a.m. – our *Love Island* schedule meant very early starts! I am learning my lines while Billy paints. He always has his brushes and art kit with him wherever he travels.

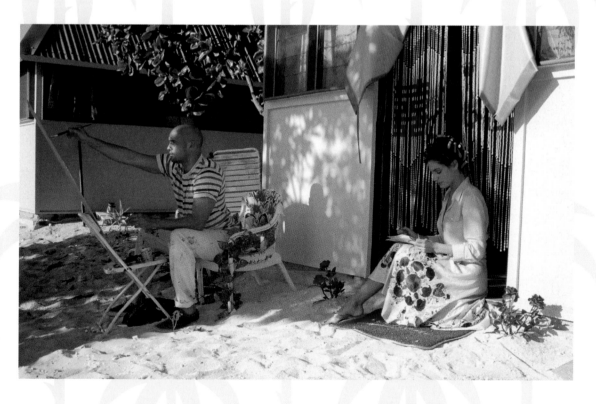

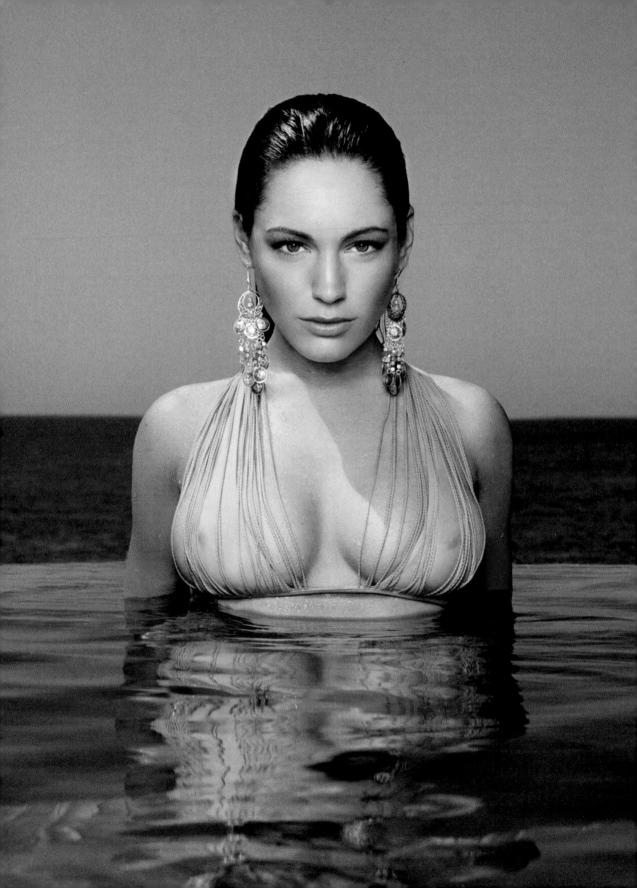

my life in the lads' mags

08

When I arrived back in England after filming *Celebrity Love Island*, I was told that readers of *FHM* magazine had voted me Sexiest Woman in the World 2005. I'd been working with *FHM* since 1997 and had become one of their regular cover girls, but it was a huge honour to be voted sexiest woman in the world, especially when I saw all the other gorgeous girls on the list! The so-called lads' mags have played a huge part in my career, and I often did photo shoots with *FHM*, *Arena*, *GQ* – I won GQ Woman of the Year while I was presenting *The Big Breakfast* – *Maxim* and *Loaded* that required me to wear very little and basically fulfil some kind of male fantasy.

My ensemble could range from wearing simple cotton bra and briefs sets with barely there make-up for a wholesome, virginal look to full-on bondage gear with all the accessories.

My first fetish-style shoot was for the specialist magazine *Skin Two*, with the photographer Perou. A company called House of Harlot had made various rubber suits, and I recall having to sprinkle whole containers full of talc inside them just to get them on! I loved dressing up as the different characters – we did a 'secretary', a 'police officer' and a 'nurse', and the pictures eventually appeared in *Rolling Stone* magazine.

I also did a fabulous shoot in various black PVC ensembles, with really sleek, shiny, poker-straight hair, with the cult portrait photographer Rankin for *Arena*, which was a more sophisticated take on the fetish theme. He later went on to do an official portrait of Her Majesty Queen Elizabeth II, but I think it's safe to say that she wore a slightly different outfit to the ones I modelled for him!

There was a time, not so long ago, when this kind of imagery would never have appeared in a mainstream magazine but would be relegated to the 'top shelf'. It's so much more acceptable now that all sorts of high-profile women, from soap stars to aristocracy, are happy to appear in risqué shoots, and even artistic fashion and portrait photographers work for the lads' mags.

left: This shoot to celebrate my being voted Sexiest Woman in the World 2005 by *FHM* readers took place in Cabo San Lucus, Mexico.

To commemorate me winning the Sexiest Woman in the World title, *FHM* flew me out to Cabo San Lucas in Mexico to do the cover shoot and take some pictures for inside the magazine with photographer James White. Again, I took Billy with me so we could enjoy the beautiful surroundings – it seems such a shame not to take advantage of these opportunities if your partner isn't working and is able to join you.

After checking into our hotel, Billy and I jumped in the car and headed to the famous Hotel California for dinner. I was amazed at the beauty of the rugged shoreline, and our room had a really stunning view, with a private swimming pool on the balcony. The following night, after a day shooting for *FHM*, we stayed in our room and watched *Like Water*

for Chocolate, one of the best Mexican movies ever, based on the novel by Laura Esquivel. Perfect!

While I did my pictures with James for *FHM*, Billy shot some behind-the-scenes footage on Super 8 film, which we later uploaded onto my website. It's great to be able to share those kinds of things on the internet, as it gives fans the chance to see a different side of you.

Once we'd finished the *FHM* shoot, Billy and I went off exploring, enjoying the vivid culture and landscape of our surroundings and buying up loads of Mexican calendar girl artwork. I've used these prints as a source of inspiration on a number of occasions, taking my lead from the vibrant colours and patterns when I'm putting together my own wardrobe.

"all sorts of high-profile women are happy to appear in risqué shoots"

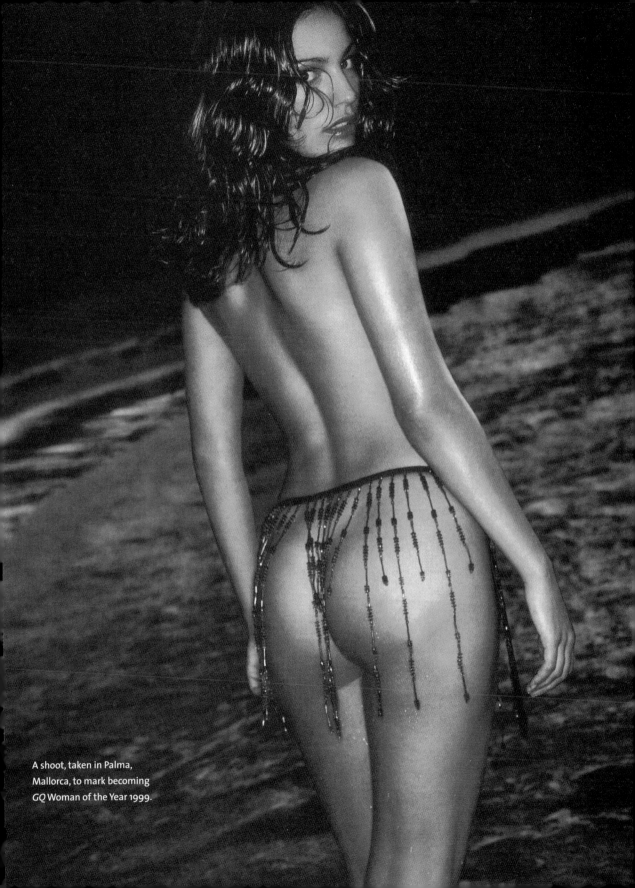

A shoot, taken in Palma,
Mallorca, to mark becoming
GQ Woman of the Year 1999.

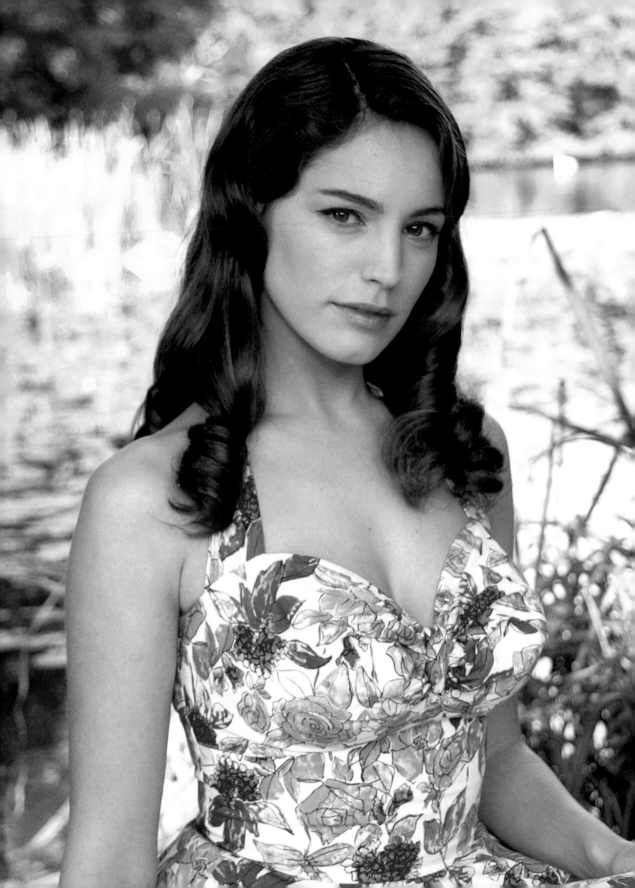

Kelly does Agatha Christie

Following my stint on *Celebrity Love Island*, an ITV executive called
Andy Harries rang to arrange a meeting to discuss other opportunities.
We met in London one day with my agent, Jan Croxson, and Andy
asked me what I'd like to do next. When I replied that I was keen to
do a period drama, the pair of them looked really shocked. When they
finally realised I wasn't joking, we started to discuss what kind of
thing might work.

After planting that initial seed, I received a call three months
later asking me to consider playing Elsie Holland, a young governess
in Agatha Christie's Miss Marple novel entitled *The Moving Finger*.
ITV were making a new series of their acclaimed 'Marple' drama series,
starring Geraldine McEwan as the ageing lady detective, and they
were keen for me to be involved. It was set in 1950s rural England and,
as you can imagine, I jumped at the chance to work on such a high-
profile project.

Looking at the cast list for my episode was truly humbling as
it was a role-call of talented, experienced classical actors: Ken Russell,
Frances de la Tour, Emilia Fox, Sean Pertwee, Imogen Stubbs, John
Sessions and even Harry Enfield were all scheduled to appear in
The Moving Finger. Suddenly I was nervous.

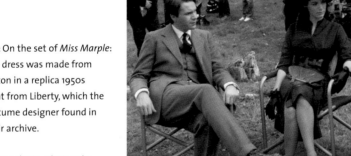

left: On the set of *Miss Marple*:
this dress was made from
cotton in a replica 1950s
print from Liberty, which the
costume designer found in
their archive.

right: Relaxing during the
filming of the Miss Marple
story *The Moving Finger*.

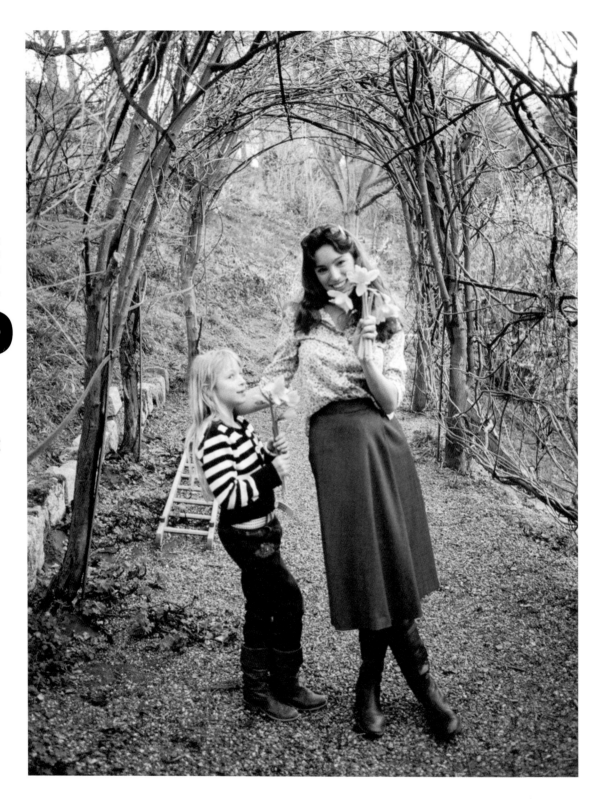

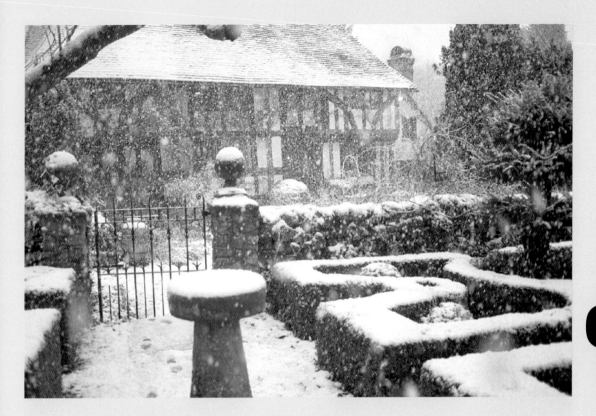

We had a wonderful costume designer on the show called Frances Tempest, who'd worked on *Calendar Girls* with Helen Mirren and Julie Walters – yes, they did wear clothes in some scenes – as well as a number of other TV and film productions. She was incredibly thorough and paid attention to the smallest details in our outfits.

We went along to the textile archive at London department store Liberty, where we ordered printed fabrics in original 1950s designs to make into sundresses and dirndl skirts, then Frances took me to a huge film and TV costume warehouse in north London, where we plundered every department for suitable attire for Elsie Holland.

I was in fashion heaven, rummaging through the rails for 1950s dresses, and trying on exquisitely elegant Ava Gardner-style picture hats. There were whole rooms filled with block-heeled shoes, and even more with seamed stockings and kid leather gloves in every colour under the sun. There were Fifties-style sunglasses and drawers bursting with costume jewellery: I felt like a little girl let loose in the world's biggest dressing-up box.

Frances insisted on me wearing authentic 1950s underwear, too, so the whole look was completely faithful to the style of the day, so I wriggled into a series of corsets, waist-cinching girdles and cone-shaped bullet bras. The shape and definition they gave my body was amazing, and they improve your posture, too – it's incredible how our casual approach to dressing has encouraged us to slouch: there's no structure to our clothing nowadays, like there used to be.

above: My house in Kent looks even more beautiful in the winter snow.

left: At home in my garden with my niece.

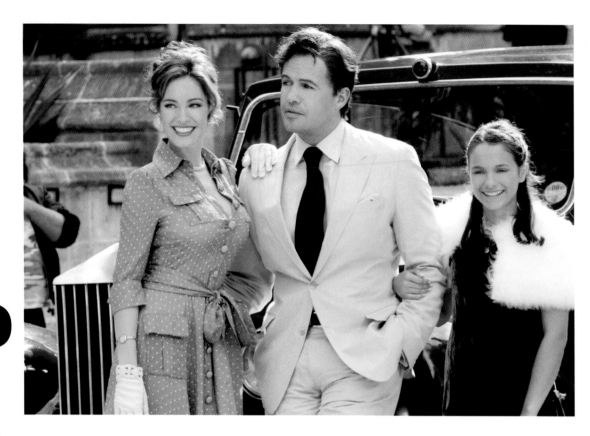

I really enjoyed the experience of wearing authentic 1950s underwear, even though it was actually very uncomfortable. It certainly exaggerated every curve on my body. I had pointy boobs and a tiny waist – no wonder all the Fifties starlets looked so fabulous wearing undergarments like that. Frances even sewed pearls into the ends of the bras, just to be extra naughty! I was so delighted with all my outfits that when shooting ended I bought every one. I just couldn't bear to part with them.

We filmed *Marple* in the English countryside, partly in the Chiltern Hills of Buckinghamshire and partly in my home territory, Kent. Having spent so much time in California before that, it really made me fall in love with England again. The rolling hills, green fields, trees and chocolate-box villages made Los Angeles feel like a big, hot concrete car park in comparison.

It wasn't surprising, therefore, that in 2006 I decided to buy a property back in England, so I could spend more time near my family in the area I truly call home. While I love the glamour of life in Hollywood, there is something special about the countryside where I grew up, and being near the people I've known and loved all my life.

My parents spotted a lovely medieval farmhouse that had just come on the market near where they live, and as soon as I saw it I fell in love with it and put an offer in immediately. My new home is steeped in history, with views across the Kent countryside and lovely romantic landscaped gardens. I have apple and pear orchards, a fresh-water spring, a herb garden, and I'm in the process of planting a scented flower garden, too. And when I'm not working, I enjoy pottering outside, cooking shepherd's pie or soup in my lovely country kitchen or going for a pint in my local pub.

Soon after we finished shooting *Marple*, Billy and I flew to Los Angeles, and one weekend in January, I settled down to read a script that had been sent to Billy by a writer called Melissa Painter. *Fishtales* was an enchanting family fairytale with a mermaid as the lead role, and, as a confirmed romantic, it captured my imagination immediately. Before pilot season had even begun, I felt I had found my project for 2006. I was really excited and called Melissa to organise a dinner so we could discuss the script more and have a round-table read. We gathered together various actor friends and read the script out loud together, so we could have a creative discussion about whether it had potential.

After that I felt it was definitely something I was keen to pursue, but I had to put *Fishtales* to the back of my mind as I was due to fly to London to launch my new lingerie collection for high-street store New Look. Once I'd unveiled my underwear designs to the world, which you can read about in the next chapter, Billy and I flew to the Amalfi coast of Italy for a short break. It was somewhere I'd always wanted to visit because I love the film *Only You* starring Robert Downey Jr and Marissa Tomei, which was filmed there.

When we checked into our hotel in Positano, and realised it was called La Sirenuse (The Siren), I was convinced it was a sign. There were lovely mosaics everywhere featuring mermaids, and I knew it meant I had to follow up my *Fishtales* project. However, as Billy was working on something else at the time, he suggested I took it on as my project, so I sent it to various contacts in London, including Alki David, who decided to buy the script and make the film with him directing. It was both nerve-racking and exciting trying to secure the funding, but by the time the Cannes Film Festival came around in May, we'd got the money we needed to make the film.

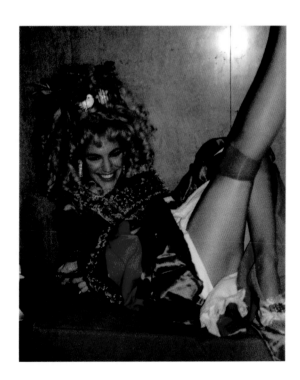

above left: Me with Billy and Amber Savva on location in London during the filming of *Fishtales*.

right: I recently appeared in an episode of the TV series *Hotel Babylon*, based on the book by Imogen Edwards-Jones. It was fun to dress up in period costume for a masked ball scene, complete with panniered, corseted dresses and pastel-coloured wigs!

Alki has a beautiful home on the Greek island of Spetses and we decided to use this as the location for the film. Billy and I travelled out early in the summer to scout for suitable coves and settings for the different scenes, and had a lovely time planning our first proper production together. We were going to play the lead roles, and we stayed with a lovely family called the Orloffs, who made us incredibly welcome for the duration of the production.

I was looking forward to my Esther Williams moment, wearing a mermaid's tail, and had commissioned an Australian special-effects team to make two tails for the project, which they had to transport all the way from Down Under. We agreed to meet at Alki's house so I could try out the tails in his swimming pool.

I had swum once before with a free diver's fin, but this was going to require a very different technique and I was quite apprehensive about swimming with a huge mermaid's tail encasing my legs. I was surprised how quickly I got the hang of it, though, and it soon began to feel quite natural, using the tail to propel me through the water.

Indeed, once I'd got used to moving through the water with my tail, it felt fairly easy, and when I first tried swimming normally, after I'd taken it off, it felt quite odd. After that, the hardest thing was learning to hold my breath long enough to film a couple of the underwater scenes. Fortunately, I had a stunt double – Hannah – who is an incredibly talented free diver who can hold her breath for much longer than me.

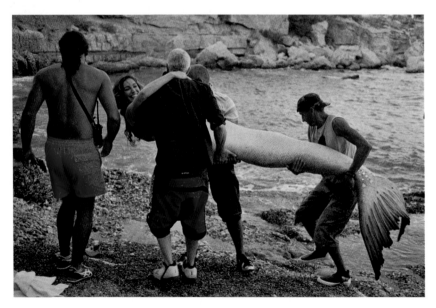

left: Being carried out of the sea during the filming of *Fishtales*, which had its UK cinema release in August 2007.

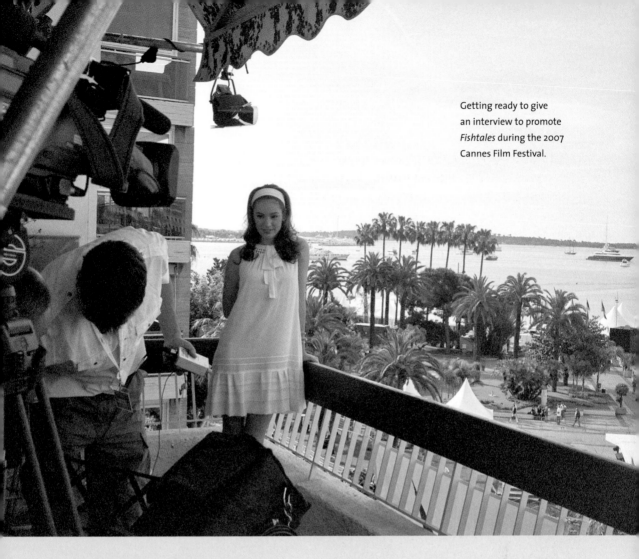

Getting ready to give
an interview to promote
Fishtales during the 2007
Cannes Film Festival.

The experience of making *Fishtales* was one that Billy and I will cherish: we were in one of our favourite parts of the world, and it was the first time we had seen a production through from start to finish, taking a script, securing funding, putting together a team and working on the project – in front of the camera as well as behind the scenes – ready for it to be edited. Alki David then worked on all the post-production and put together his vision of the film to the point where it was ready to show the rest of the world.

In May 2007, Billy and I took the final cut to the Cannes Film Festival for its first screening to the press and the big players in terms of distribution, which is always a nerve-racking experience. We did the usual photocalls (remember Brigitte Bardot's famous Cannes photocalls? It's all part of the theatre of the Film Festival) and networked with all the right people. Thankfully, we secured a great distribution deal with Showcase Cinemas in the UK and across Europe, and the film was released in August 2007, so we had a happy ending to our mermaid's tale (or should I say 'tail'?!).

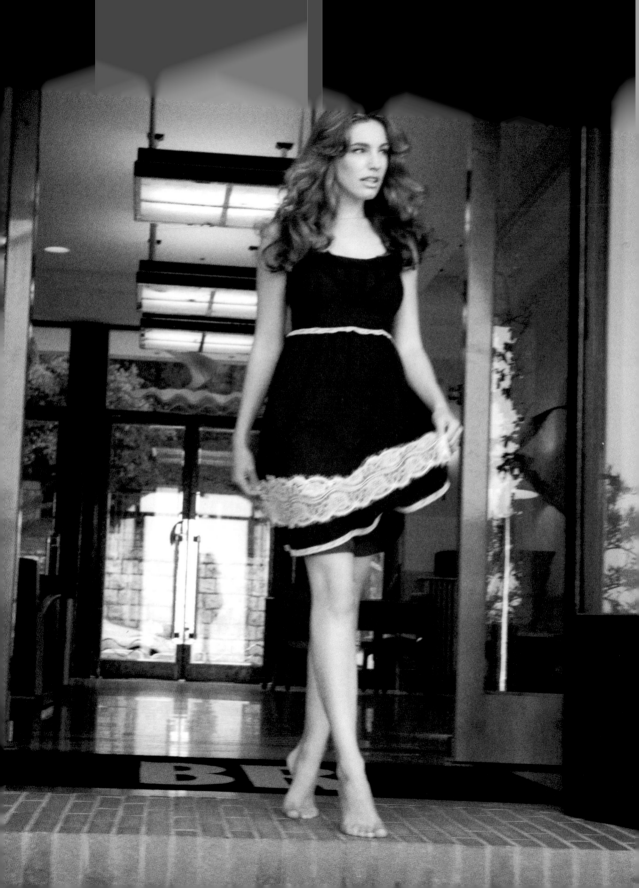

10

Kelly Brook: the brand

For many years, I've harboured a secret desire to design my own lingerie and swimwear collections. I've worn so many different shapes and styles over the years that I have very strong opinions about what works and what doesn't, and have struggled to find brands that cater for my personal taste. I've even had to resort to having things made up to my own specifications, and when I've worn them, people love them.

In the last ten years, I've seen a huge boom in the choice that women have. When I started modelling, it was really hard to find stylish swimwear and underwear if you were anything other than an average 34B, and when you did find something pretty, it usually required a mortgage to buy it. Even my smaller-busted friends have benefited from the array of different brands that have launched in the last decade. But I still felt there was something missing: something feminine and flattering, fun and sexy, with the old-fashioned glamour of a bygone era, and the fit and function of contemporary fabrics and manufacturing.

For a while I'd felt there was a gap in the market for someone to create and sell the sort of styles I love, and I'd been toying with my own designs. So, in the summer of 2005, after I returned from filming *Celebrity Love Island* in Fiji, I met with a licensing company in London who I'd previously had tentative discussions with about launching a branded collection of swimwear.

Inspired by the pieces I'd worn on *Love Island*, I had done some preliminary sketches and gathered together some visuals and samples that I felt represented the sort of look I aimed to achieve. I wanted a vintage feel, with flirty pin-up-inspired styling, but they had to work with the modern woman's lifestyle. We looked at pictures of Brigitte Bardot and Marilyn Monroe, as well as photos of me wearing original 1950s pieces in Fiji. We met up with a licensing manager, who loved the idea, so I set to work on my first collection. After two months, I'd developed a range of designs I was pleased with – now it was time to find a retailer to partner me on the collection.

I was determined that if I were to put the range into production, it would have to be available in a broad range of sizes to accommodate the needs of different-shaped women, and would have to be priced at accessible levels. I wanted people to be able to afford to buy the Kelly Brook collection, not to feel it was out of reach.

I had a number of meetings with different retailers, many of whom expressed an interest in working with me, but it was New Look who I felt offered the right home for my product. They seemed the best commercial match for a number of reasons: they have over 700 stores and plans to expand into Europe, which obviously meant there was potential for really good distribution, and hopefully good sales, too. But the thing that helped secure the New Look contract for me was the diversity of their customer base. They catered for different ages, from teenage shoppers to older women, and varying sizes, which was exactly the idea behind my range. The deal was done: Kelly Brook at New Look.

It was incredibly exciting to be developing a whole creative concept alongside the product range, and I had all sorts of ideas for labelling, point-of-sale material and publicity shots, but I needed someone I trusted to bring them to life. When you're putting your name to something that you've devoted so much time and energy to, it's really important to have the team you want on board – for example, I've always worked with the photographer Alan Strutt on my calendar, because he knows me so well that he has an almost instinctive feel for what I'm trying to achieve creatively.

I've long admired the work of Paul Solomon, the art director at *GQ* magazine: he's always had fantastically inspiring ideas for photographic shoots, and I felt he was the man to translate my name into a sexy, commercial brand identity that would sell. So Paul and I had an initial chat about the concept behind the collection, and we bounced around some ideas for photography and branding. He was keen to get a photographer called Simon Emmett to shoot the publicity shots that would accompany the launch of Kelly Brook at New Look, and presented me with a creative proposal I instantly loved, though I was intrigued to see how it would be achieved.

On the day of the shoot, when I arrived at the photographic studio, I was greeted by a vast water tank and scaffold structure. Paul had commissioned it, and the idea was that Simon would take his shots *through* the water, with me suspended in different positions behind the tank, so it looked like I was in the water. It was all an optical illusion, as the reality of creating beautiful pictures underwater is very tough. This way, we could control hair and make-up, and achieve a glamorous Esther Williams-inspired set of pictures.

The shoot took nine hours, after which Simon and Paul had got what they set out to achieve, and I was thrilled with the results. My vision for the Kelly Brook brand was starting to become a reality.

right: One of the stunning shots taken to launch my New Look swimwear collection.

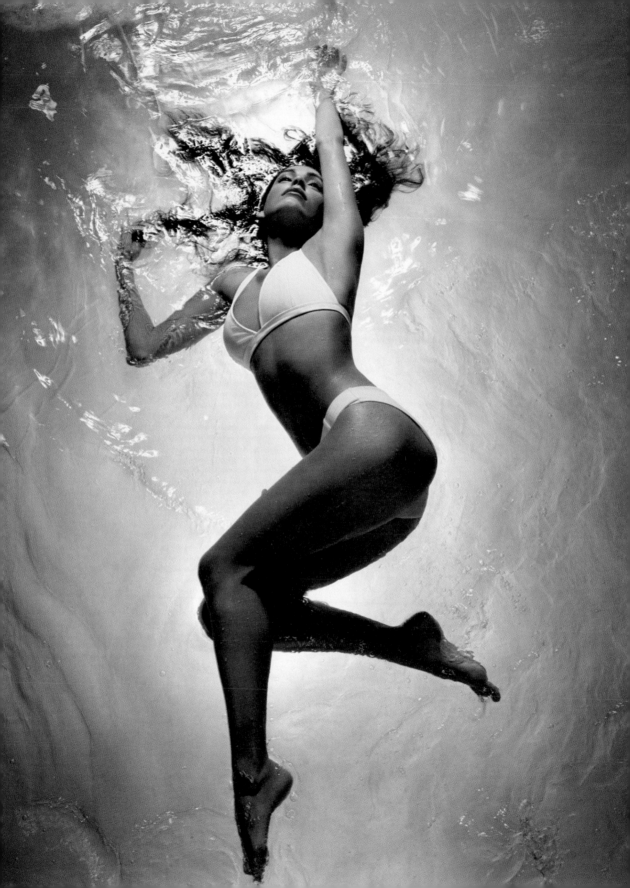

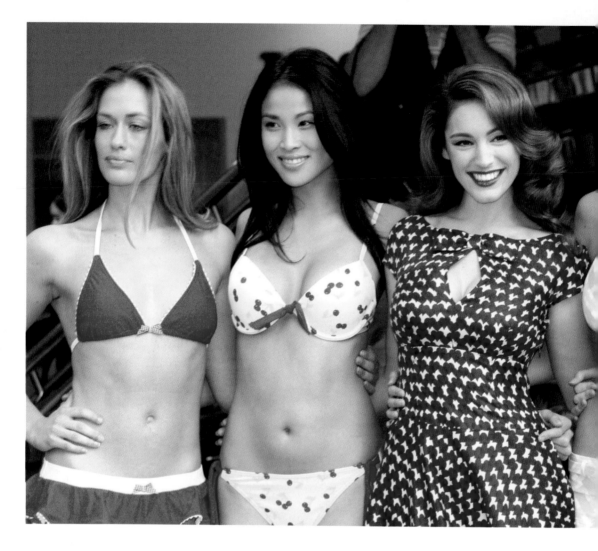

In April 2006, we launched the Kelly Brook at New Look swimwear collection with a whistlestop tour of London, Glasgow and Dublin, all in one day. I flew by private jet, accompanied by four models wearing bikinis from the collection – I felt like Hugh Hefner and his playgirls! I did personal appearances in-store, signed autographs, posed for photographs with fans and did media interviews and press photocalls. It was a great day, because it was the first time I saw my brand displayed in a retail environment.

I was amazed when I saw the papers the next day as there were pictures everywhere, and the reviews of the range were really positive. I couldn't believe that the girl everyone wrote off after *The Big Breakfast* was once again in the spotlight, being fêted as an influential style icon.

The proof of the pudding is always in the eating, though, and it was no good having acres of media coverage if my designs didn't sell. And only time would tell if the collection was a commercial success.

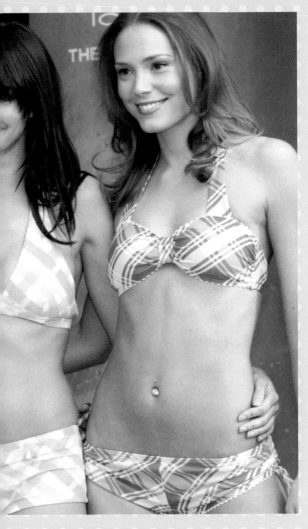

left: At the launch of my first
swimwear collection for New
Look in April 2006. Although I'm
not wearing a bikini myself, this
is one of my favourite 'bikini
moments' – I was really proud to
launch my collection, but didn't
want to model the range myself
that day as I wanted to be
perceived as the businesswoman
behind the brand, not just the
body.

I waited in a state of anxious trepidation for the first set of sales figures to come through from the buyers at New Look. One minute I was petrified the range would be a flop, the next I was confidently predicting that people would love it, but no one was more surprised – and delighted – than me when the call came through to say that sales were 80 per cent above predictions! The team at New Look was over the moon and I was ecstatic, so we immediately begin discussing what we could do next ...

After the runaway success of my first foray into fashion design, New Look felt confident in me as a commercial prospect and asked if I'd be interested in creating an own-label lingerie collection to complement the swimwear range. This, of course, was a dream come true for me, and I immediately started work, creating the kind of lingerie I love to wear.

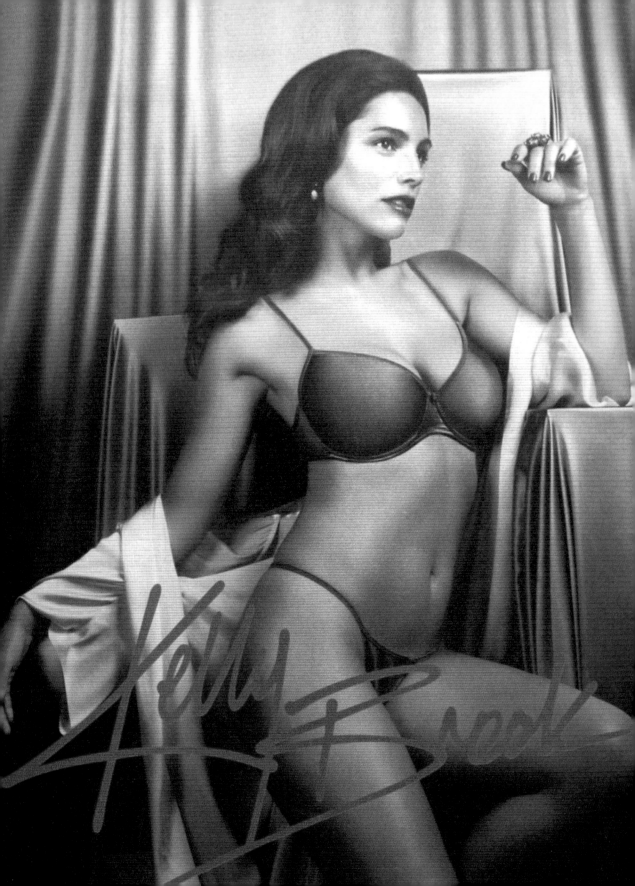

I wanted to design pieces that were not only gorgeous to look at, in a subtle, elegant colour palette, but that were tactile, too, made from beautiful silks and good-quality lace. Most of all I felt it was imperative that the bras gave the structure and support necessary to give a woman the best shape possible, regardless of whether she's a B-cup or an E-cup. Whatever size you are, there's a bra style that will enhance your curves, and I wanted to provide enough variety in the collection to offer something for everyone.

Not long before I started working on the lingerie collection, I went to an exhibition at London's Royal Academy of Arts which had really inspired me. Maria Górska was born in 1898, the daughter of a wealthy Polish lawyer and his socialite wife, and she spent her childhood at boarding school in Switzerland, holidaying with her grandmother in Italy and on the French Riviera. She married young, at just eighteen, and settled in Russia, but a year later she moved with her husband, Tadeusz Lempicki, to Paris, where she gave herself a new name: Tamara de Lempicka.

During the 1920s, Tamara de Lempicka studied art and began mixing with the bohemian crowd in Paris, counting Pablo Picasso and Jean Cocteau among her friends. Her portraits rapidly gained a reputation, and throughout the 1930s she was considered one of the world's most innovative artists. Today, Madonna and Jack Nicholson are collectors of her Art Deco-influenced work.

Witnessing the dramatic style of de Lempicka's striking figurative paintings was a revelation to me: I'd never seen women depicted as such strong and beautiful creatures. I loved the way she made her subjects look so powerful, without underplaying their voluptuous curves and feminine charms. I also loved her unusual use of colour: the cool steel blues with the rich, deep russet browns; the pale fleshy tones contrasting with rosebud lips in shocking scarlet; the gun-metal greys paired with rich emerald greens.

left: Tamara de Lempicka inspired the advertising campaign for my New Look lingerie range.

I had unwittingly found my starting point for the Kelly Brook at New Look lingerie line: the work of Tamara de Lempicka. I began collecting together all the material I could find: books, postcards, posters and pieces of fabric that resembled the feel I was hoping for. The range was due to launch ready for the Christmas 2006 season, and I wanted it to be grown-up, sophisticated and sensual, like Lempicka's paintings.

Then I sat down with the in-house design team at New Look and we set to work. It's incredible how much work goes into the design and manufacturing process of any garment, but a bra, in particular, is incredibly complex. It can feature dozens of components and is effectively a piece of engineering, rather than dressmaking. I think perhaps my dad, as an experienced scaffolder, might have been a better bra designer than my grandmother, who was a talented seamstress!

I learned so much about the difficulties – or should I say challenges? – facing designers when they are trying to create an attractive bra. Fabrics have to be strong enough to withstand tension, but most of us prefer the material used to feel soft and flimsy, and materials that look fabulous as a sample might not work as well in the four-inch square piece that's required to create a bra cup.

Though it was a steep learning curve, I had a very strong idea of the look I wanted to create, and I worked very closely with the designers to achieve this. When it came to selecting fabrics, they respected my choices, though on one occasion I had to fight very hard for what I wanted.

I was really keen to have a leopard-print element to the collection, but Sharon, the buyer, insisted that animal prints never sell. She was adamant that it would be commercial suicide, but I practically got down on my knees and begged her, and she eventually allowed me to include it in the range. She did, though, take some persuading.

In the end my instincts were right: around the time of the launch, Kate Moss was photographed wearing a leopard-print dress, and suddenly everyone was clamouring for animal prints, and we looked like the ones with our finger on the fashion pulse. Retailers spend thousands of pounds trying to forecast trends, but sometimes I think you just have to go with your intuition: wear what you like, and if it works, others might follow. I think that's why Kate Moss has been so influential, and in an odd way, my range benefited from her going against the fashion grain.

When I suggested including leopard print in the range, it wasn't because I was trying to predict fashion; I just love it: it's alluring and adds a feline element to any seduction. I had a gut instinct that others would share my passion for animal magic, and in the end, it became one of the collection's bestsellers. Although who knows if Sharon would have been proved right had Kate not worn her Lanvin leopard-print number?

Retail trade was very slow in the lead-up to Christmas that year, and economists kept saying that shoppers were staying away from the high street, but when New Look announced their figures were up by 4 per cent, and the *Daily Telegraph* put a photo of me on the front page of their business section, attributing this upturn to 'new brands', it was possibly the proudest moment of my career. What had started as a frivolous idea – playing 'dress-up' and wanting to design my own collection just like all little girls dream of doing – had turned into a viable venture.

All the hard work had paid off and Kelly Brook is now a successful, profitable brand. So what would I do next? I had a number of ideas, but the one at the forefront of my mind was the idea of creating a signature fragrance. When I was a little girl, I would spend sunny summer afternoons in my parents' garden plucking rose petals from their thorny stems and mixing them with water to make my own home-made perfumes.

When Bayliss and Harding suggested I meet with their beauty division to discuss the idea of developing a beauty range, I leapt at the idea. My first instinct was to suggest a fragrance, which they agreed had lots of potential, so they arranged for me to spend a day at the UK's top perfume house, CPL Aromas in Bishop's Stortford. Based in a stunning stately home in the Hertfordshire countryside, the 'noses' – trained fragrance experts who have a very highly developed sense of smell – at CPL have worked with brands like Nicole Farhi, Jasper Conran and Agent Provocateur to create just the right scent to encapsulate the personality of the label.

I had no idea how the process of creating a perfume worked, but I'd done some background research on the ingredients of my favourite perfumes, as well as making notes on smells I really

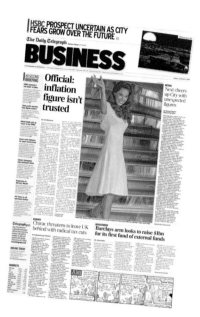

liked, and on the appointed day, a chauffeur-driven Rolls-Royce Phantom arrived to take me to their offices.

My introduction to the world of perfume was fascinating. The 'noses' explained that perfumes have a series of different 'notes' – the ingredients that are blended to create the final smell. The 'top notes' are the most prominent ingredients that hit first when you sniff a perfume, but there are 'middle notes' and 'bottom notes' too, that develop with time. This is why sometimes the character of a perfume changes a little after you first apply it. The art of creating a fragrance is very precise and the delicate balance of ingredients has to be exactly right for a scent to appeal to a commercial audience. Science was never this much fun at school!

top right: Making headlines in the business pages of the broadsheet press.

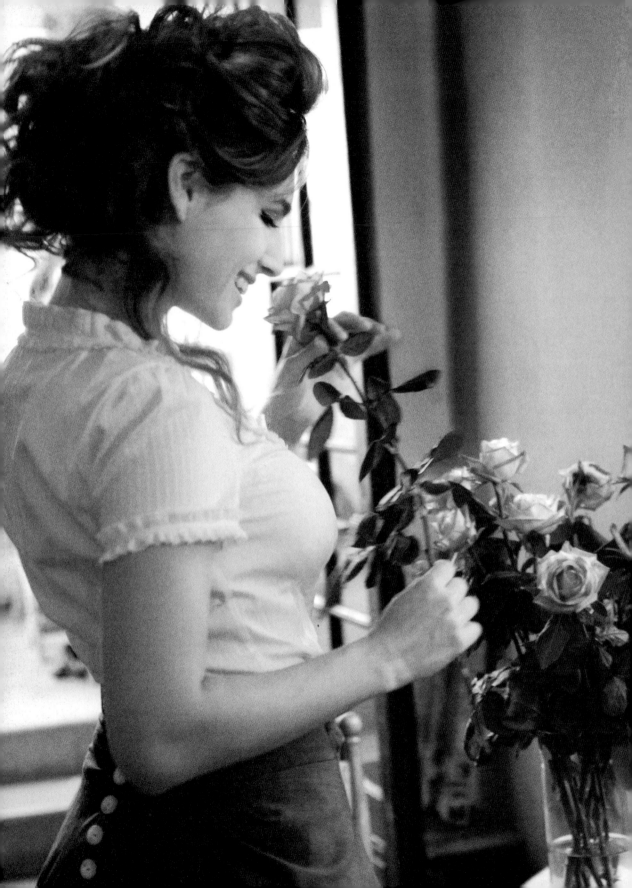

Having been briefed in advance by me and the beauty team at Bayliss and Harding, the people at CPL had created a selection of twenty-nine different blends, which they asked me to edit down to a handful of favourites. It was quite a daunting prospect, but once I'd begun, I was amazed at how easy it was to reject the ones I didn't like. It was intriguing to discover how consistent I was with my preferences: all the ones I kept had musky, vanilla top notes. Interestingly, my long-time favourite fragrance is Miranda by Fragonard, which is a musky vanilla-based scent.

I finally chose sample number twenty-seven. The CPL team were thrilled that I'd selected that one, as it's their lucky fragrance sample number, and confidently predicted that it would be a success. The experience of identifying a perfume that represents my character was one of the most enjoyable days I've ever had, and I thoroughly recommend it to anyone who has the opportunity to try it.

That night, after being driven back to London in the Rolls-Royce, we enjoyed a celebratory dinner at one of my favourite restaurants: Cipriani in Davies Street. I had a delicious white truffle risotto – what a treat! – and the team at CPL presented me with a beautiful crystal Tiffany vase as a belated birthday present. It suddenly dawned on me – I had just turned twenty-seven – now my lucky number!

As for what is next for Kelly Brook? Well, all I can say is: watch this space!

'These are a few of my favourite things'...

CAKE SHOPS
Hummingbird Bakery, Portobello Road, London
Magnolia Bakery, New York
Sprinkles Cupcakes, Los Angeles
Sweet Lady Jane, Los Angeles

LINGERIE AND DRESS-UP
Trashy Lingerie, Los Angeles
Agent Provocateur
Frederick's of Hollywood, Los Angeles
Coco de Mer, London

FAVOURITE VINTAGE BOUTIQU
The Girl Can't Help It, Alf
Divine Decadence, Taranto,
Fly Boutique, Miami, Flavic
The Way We Wore, Los Ange

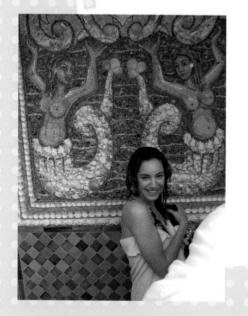

FAVOURITE MOVIE MOMENTS
James Dean and Elizabeth Taylor in Giant
Elvis Presley and Ann-Margret in Viva Las Vegas
Marilyn Monroe and Jane Russell in Gentlemen Pr
Clark Gable and Vivien Leigh in Gone with the Wind
My all-time favourite movie moment is Rita Hayu

FAVOURITE DESIGNERS
Balenciaga
Moschino
Vivienne Westwood
Christian Louboutin

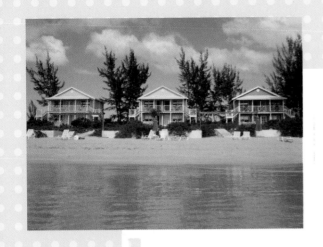

MY FAVOURITE BEACH DESTINATIONS
Byron Bay, Australia
Banyan Tree, Maldives
Molos Beach, Paros, Greece
Coco di Mama, Eleuthera, Bahamas
Shell Beach, St Barts
Croyde Bay, Cornwall

MOVIES
The Red Shoes
Singin' in the Rain

tique Market, London

HOMES FROM HOME, MY FAVOURITE HOTELS TO VISIT
The Lowell, New York
Villa Feltrinelli, Lake Garda, Italy
Hotel Bel-Air, Los Angeles
Hotel Costes, Paris
Le Sirenuse, Positano, Italy

FAVOURITE ALL-TIME TV SHOWS
I Love Lucy
The Judy Garland Show
Fame

ndes

n Gilda

Kelly x

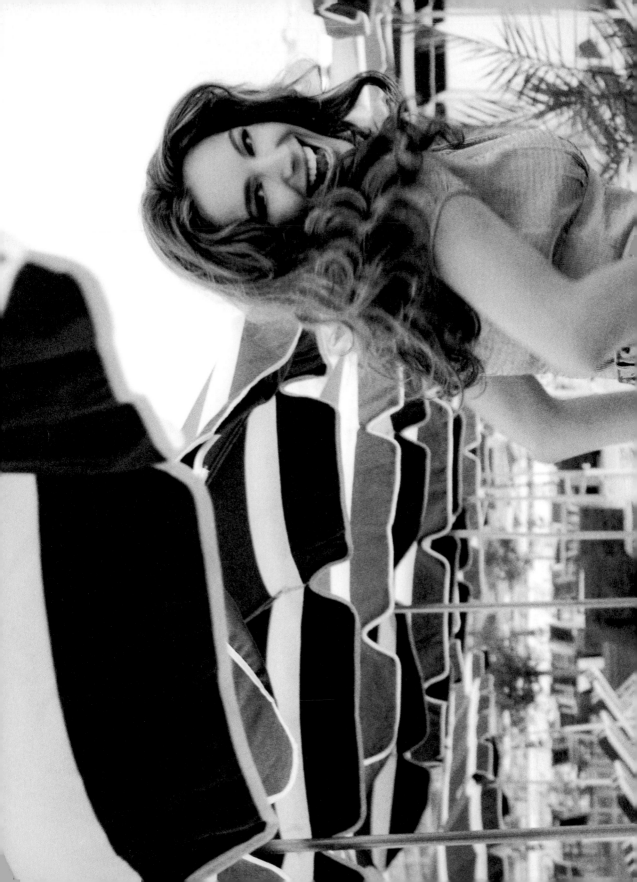

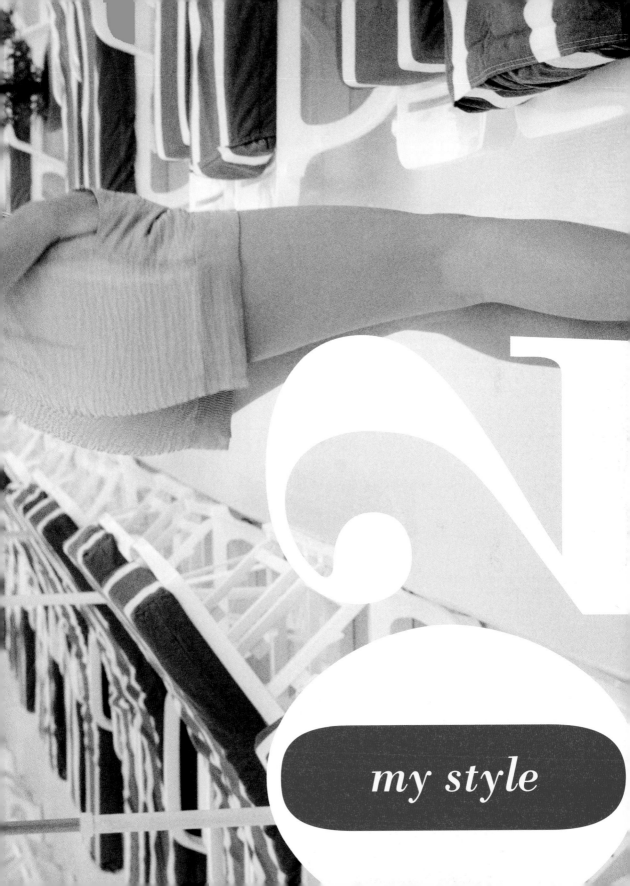

2

my style

introduction

Throughout my life I've enjoyed experimenting with different fashions and finding a style that works for me. Today, I like to think I dress to flatter my body shape, suit my lifestyle and reflect my personality. I don't profess to be a trendsetter or a fashion icon, but when my friends ask my advice on style, I think one of the most important factors is knowing yourself and having the confidence to define what works for you. It's not about following the pack, but about understanding how to draw from current and past fashions to create your own look.

I don't believe anyone has a truly original style: all of us draw inspiration, consciously or unconsciously, from our surroundings. The most avant-garde fashion designers are often found rummaging in costume archives, vintage clothing stores, thrift shops and libraries, searching for another look to reinvent. When their creations become truly original, they're usually also unwearable, because, let's face it, there's only so much you can do to clothe the human body in a practical way – and most of it's been done before.

Even the most influential trendsetters today pull their look together using vintage pieces as the basis for their style. So there's no shame in utilising retro fashion as a starting point for your look – just make sure you identify the shapes and styles that work for you, and put them together so you don't look like you've walked straight off a period drama set.

Likewise, if you admire the way certain people dress, don't be afraid to use them as inspiration when you're compiling your own wardrobe – just don't clone their look completely. As a young girl, as I've already said, I was greatly influenced by Madonna, and used to dress in copycat clothes, faithfully mimicking every last detail, from the lace fingerless gloves and leggings to the crucifix jewellery. Today, I like to think I have a slightly more subtle approach to using external references to create a look.

I love the 1950s because it's an era where women dressed demurely without losing their feminine allure: it was a period of sensual style, where curves were celebrated and womanliness was accentuated. And although many view the period as one where women were portrayed as subservient domestic goddesses, who weren't liberated until the 1960s and 1970s, I think there is something empowering about choosing to celebrate your femininity in the twenty-first century.

In our post-feminist society, you can still enjoy independent views and carve your own niche in the world, without losing sight of those assets that make you who you are. After all, when was a man afraid to show off his testosterone-fuelled character?

So much of the Kelly Brook style is influenced by the fashions of the Fifties that I wanted to outline how different elements from that period have helped shape the style I have today. I haven't set out to be a carbon copy of a certain starlet, or to replicate the designer styles of the day, but I have used the mood of the time as a starting point to build my own style.

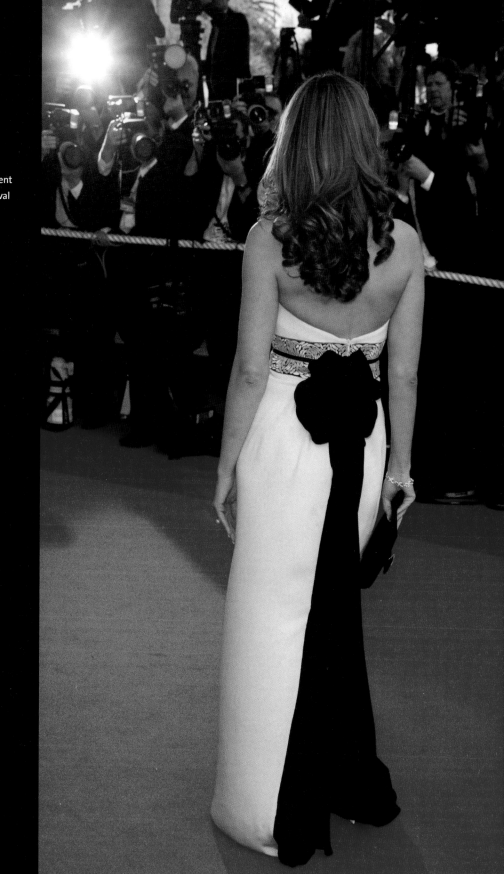

right: A red carpet moment at the Cannes Film Festival in 2007.

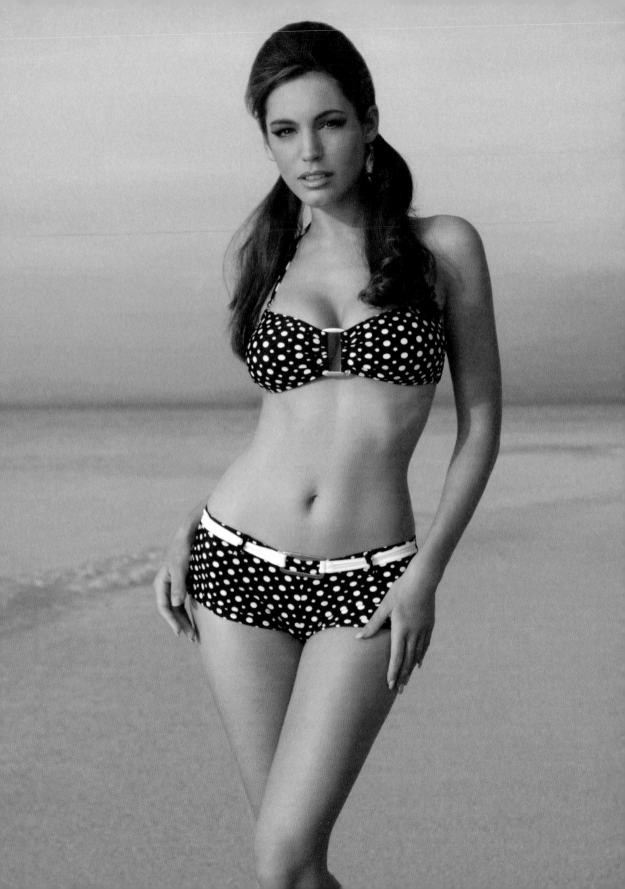

my pin-ups

11

For as long as I can remember, I have looked to the pin-up girls of the mid-twentieth century as a benchmark of female gorgeousness. Although they are usually seen as idealised versions of womanhood, the poster girls often portray an attainable glamour achieved through grooming, the choice of beautiful clothes and a confident, sexy smile.

Whether they were photographs of high-profile models and actresses who were considered sex symbols, such as Brigitte Bardot, Marilyn Monroe or Doris Day, or the stylised illustrations popularised by artists such as Alberto Vargas or Merlin Enabnit, the pin-up girls brought feminine beauty to the masses, from the 1940s onwards, in the form of postcards, posters and calendars.

One of the early pin-up girls was actress Betty Grable, whose photograph adorned the locker of many a homesick – and lovesick – GI during the Second World War. Over the years there have been a number of women who've become legendary pin-ups, or 'cheesecake girls' as they're sometimes known.

The following women are some of those who have inspired me over the years. You should make your own list of women who you feel can help guide your own design ideas, or whose body shape is similar to your own.

left: I love the retro style of this bikini, which I could imagine being worn by many of my pin-ups.

Bettie Page

Bettie Page was raised in Nashville, Tennessee, by a mother who didn't want her and a father who molested her. Growing up in immense poverty, she was a bright student and always had a sweet smile on her face as she dreamed of stardom. As a teenager, she moved to New York and began posing as a model for amateur photographers, who adored the uninhibited way she would smile provocatively, with smouldering eyes, her decency rarely covered.

Bettie Page seemed to take great joy in working as one of the early glamour models and did so with great success for about seven years from 1950. However, the resulting 'pin-up' photographs were considered offensive by many. The authorities suggested she was violating a number of sexual taboos and brought a United States Senate Committee investigation against her.

Thank goodness those attitudes didn't exist when I began glamour modelling or I'd be in the same boat!

Suddenly, she became 'the notorious Bettie Page' and disappeared almost overnight. No one knew what had become of her. Rumours and conspiracy theories abounded, but the legend lived on, with a growing fan base who adored this most playful of poster girls. For four decades she remained in hiding, and today she remains an elusive figure. When anyone recognises her and asks if she is Bettie, she apparently responds, 'Who's that?'

For me, Bettie Page has been a huge inspiration. She seemed to have so much fun posing for the camera, no matter how naughty her poses or how little she was wearing. The fact that she was smiling or laughing so genuinely made what were essentially controversial images feel harmless. I think she had a very healthy attitude, one that many modern women could learn from: she enjoyed being a woman and was completely at ease with her body and her sexuality.

" the Queen of the
of the century, yo
one of its best ke

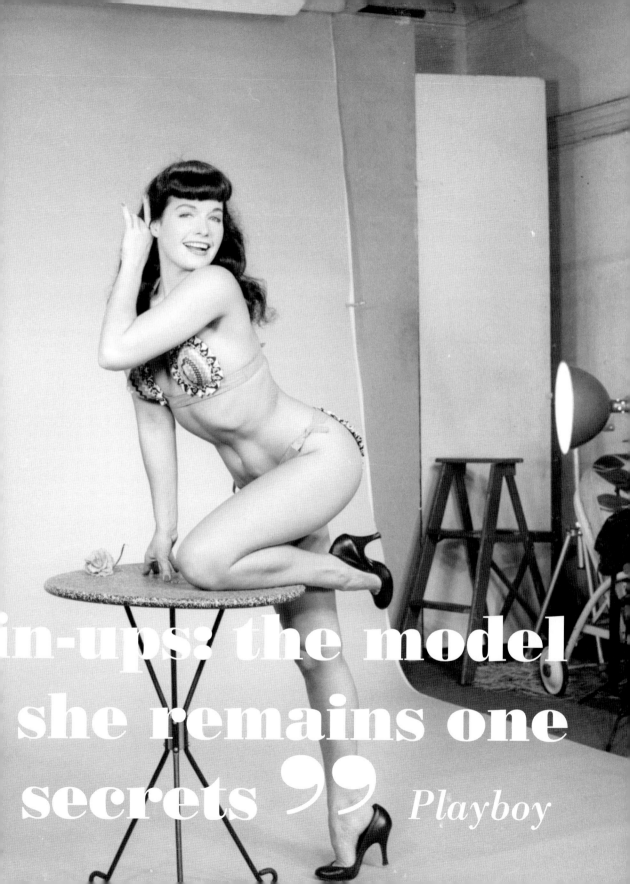

in-ups: the model she remains one secrets 99 *Playboy*

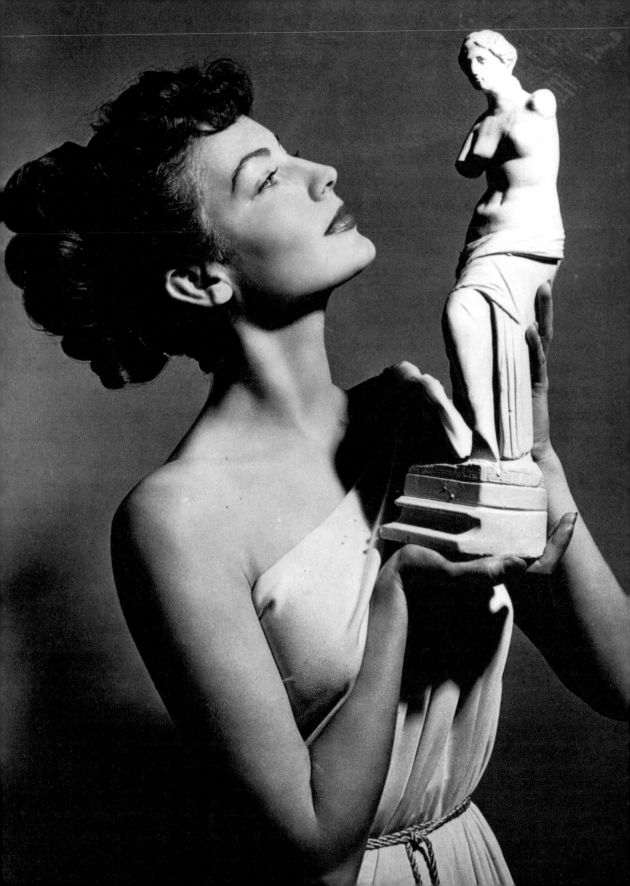

Ava Gardner

Ava Lavinia Gardner, the youngest of seven children, was born on Christmas Eve 1922 in North Carolina, where she was recognised for her classical beauty even as a child. After graduating from high school and completing a secretarial course, Ava travelled to New York City one summer to visit her elder sister, Bappie, and her husband Larry, who worked as a professional photographer. He took a number of pictures of his seventeen-year-old sister-in-law and displayed one of them in the window of his studio.

A passer-by suggested Larry forward the photographs to MGM, which he duly did, and Ava was summoned for a screen test. She signed a contract with the Hollywood studio in 1941, and Bappie acted as chaperone to her younger sister, travelling to the west coast with her and assisting in the management of her career.

Though she went on to be a leading lady opposite the likes of Burt Lancaster, Gregory Peck and Clark Gable – she gained an Oscar nomination for her role opposite him in *Mogambo* – Gardner was really cast into the spotlight as a result of her high-profile marriages to Mickey Rooney, band-leader Artie Shaw and blue-eyed boy Frank Sinatra, which was described by *People* magazine as one of the 'romances of the century'. They were married in 1951 and divorced five years later, unable to survive the demands of their dual careers and their obsessive jealousy of each other.

To many, however, Ava's biggest asset was her serene, sensual beauty: she wasn't brazenly sexy, but she was alluring in an aloof way. She had a detached charm that set her apart as a perfect being. In *One Touch of Venus* she looks divine in a gorgeous white Grecian gown, playing a statue of the goddess Venus that comes to life. She could carry off an array of necklines – sweetheart, one-shouldered, square, strapless and off-the-shoulder – and always looked fabulous. And she knew how to work a jumper, too. She was, in my eyes, the ultimate sweater girl.

left: Ava Gardner had a classical beauty that was perfectly illustrated in *One Touch of Venus*.

Sophia Loren

Sofia Scicolone was born in Rome in 1934, and raised by her unmarried mother, who struggled to feed and clothe her young daughter. Sofia spent much of her childhood witnessing the horrors of the Second World War first hand, suffering a shrapnel wound to her chin when she was just six years old.

Five years later, when peace was declared and the local theatre reopened, Sofia would spend hours watching her favourite Hollywood stars on the big screen, including Clark Gable, Cary Grant, Rita Hayworth, June Allyson and Betty Grable. She would often stay for three or four screenings in a row, dreaming of one day being a film star herself, just like I did as a child. And just like me, Sofia's body turned from that of a child into that of a woman very quickly in her early teens.

At the age of fourteen, her mother entered her in a beauty contest in Naples, despite protestations from her daughter and the lower age limit being fifteen. Sofia found herself one of the twelve princesses attending the newly crowned Queen of the Sea. This early success in beauty pageants encouraged Sofia to take acting classes, and alongside her growing reputation in beauty contests, she quickly made a name for herself as an extra in a number of film productions. Her first audition saw her cast as a slave girl in the Mervyn LeRoy film, *Quo Vadis*. She later changed her name to Sophia Loren and went on to work opposite many of the silver screen legends she had admired as a child, such as Cary Grant, Frank Sinatra and Clark Gable.

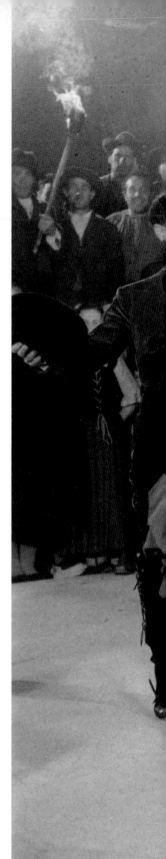

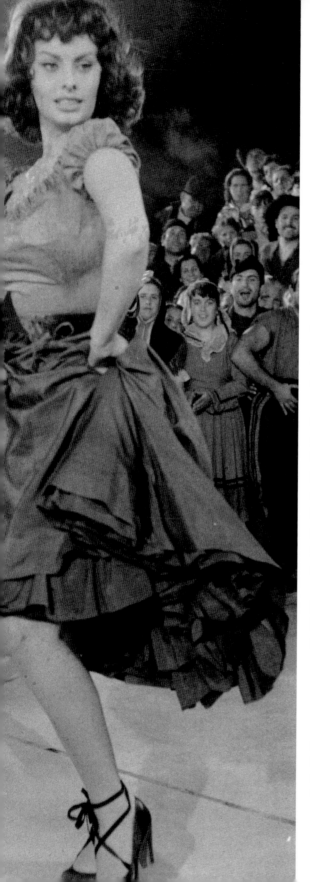

I love the romance of Sophia Loren's life story: the way she fulfilled her childhood ambitions and more. She also epitomises the grown-up, groomed goddess-like glamour I've always aspired to. She has an almost untouchable quality and an incredible sense of her own identity, despite being pressured during her acting career to diet and have plastic surgery – critics of her early screen tests suggested her nose was too long and her hips too large: what did they know?! She was content with the body Mother Nature gave her and became a sex symbol on her own terms.

I look at many of her early pictures today and think how timeless her style was: those gorgeous dresses that caressed her curves would be just as relevant now as they were in the 1950s. Even as an older woman today, she exudes a sensual allure that's elegant and refined. She knows what suits her and presents herself accordingly – the striking cats'-eye make-up and the pale pouting lips, the curvy silhouette and neat, artfully styled coiffure.

What I think any woman can learn from Sophia Loren is that even if some aspects of your looks aren't deemed to be 'right', you can still be beautiful if that's how you feel.

left: Sophia Loren's dramatic looks weren't initially to everyone's tastes, but even now she exudes a sensual allure.

" nothing makes a woman more beautiful than the belief that she is beautiful "

Sophia Loren

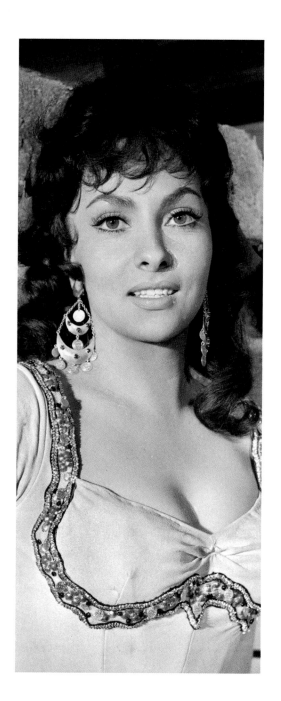

Gina Lollobrigida

Luigina Lollobrigida was born in 1927, and grew up in a small Italian mountain village, but found herself propelled into the world of beauty pageants and modelling from an early age. At the age of three she had already been voted the 'most beautiful child in Italy', and as a teenager she took small parts in Italian films. By the time she was twenty she had come third in the Miss Italy beauty contest, showing that winning beauty pageants is a well-trodden path into acting for Hollywood starlets!

In 1953, the woman who by then was known as Gina Lollobrigida appeared in her first Hollywood production, and two years later she appeared in the aptly titled film *The World's Most Beautiful Woman*.

'Lollo' was an Italian sensation, fêted in her homeland for her beauty, and I have long been a fan. As a young woman she had a bewitching charm that must have seduced many male admirers. She didn't have the voluptuous curves of Sophia Loren, but she dressed to enhance her femininity, with neat, fitted sweaters, corseted dresses, dramatic colours and exotic jewellery. I loved the way she wore huge gypsy-style hoop earrings, which I've adopted on occasion, too.

With her unique style, Gina ensured she stood out from the rest and did it so well that she won many admirers, and this is another tip we can all learn from: to create our own look, and not feel constrained by the norms of fashion.

left: Gina Lollobrigida's unique style and 'gypsy' ear-rings won her fans around the world.

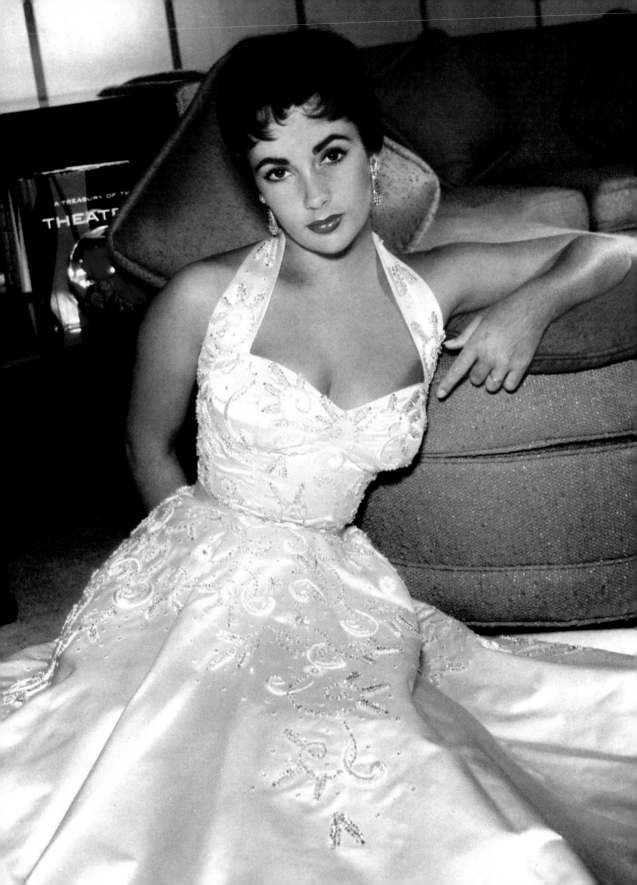

Elizabeth Taylor

When I was growing up in Kent, I used to watch Elizabeth Taylor films on Sunday afternoons and be entranced by her exquisite beauty and glamour. Her bewitching violet eyes are some of the most striking I've ever seen, framed – apparently blessed by a freak of nature – by a double row of eyelashes. She was the epitome of womanhood: a super-elegant, silver-screen version of my grandmother in the wedding portrait that sat in our living room.

Born in Hampstead, north London, in 1932 to American parents, Elizabeth took her first ballet lessons at the age of three, then, when the Second World War broke out four years later, her mother moved the family to Los Angeles to avoid the hostilities. By 1941, a nine-year-old Elizabeth had already appeared in her first feature film, but it was in the 1943 *Lassie Come Home* that she was to enjoy her first taste of stardom.

A year later, at the age of twelve, Taylor starred opposite Mickey Rooney in the blockbuster *National Velvet*, playing Velvet Brown, a young girl who trains her horse to run in – and win – the Grand National. She went on to win two Oscars, appearing in classic films such as *Cleopatra*, when she first met Richard Burton, who played Mark Antony, and *Cat on a Hot Tin Roof* opposite Paul Newman.

I'm entranced by Elizabeth Taylor who, though her health has deteriorated, still exudes an unmistakable star quality. She has enjoyed a decadent lifestyle, famously adoring diamond jewellery and accruing a number of extravagant pieces from her various husbands.

In her youth, she epitomised classical beauty, and was a woman who was blessed with perfect features and the talent to go with it.

left: Elizabeth Taylor was always one of the most stylish Hollywood icons.

Jayne Mansfield

As a child of five, Vera Jayne Palmer would put on theatrical performance for anyone who would watch, which was usually her menagerie of cuddly animals, which I can relate to! And as she grew older, she would play the violin on her parents' front lawn for passers-by.

When Vera was thirteen years old, she visited the Twentieth Century Fox Studios in Hollywood with her mother. Legend has it that afterwards the pair of them were sitting having lunch in a local diner when the teenager spotted two radio stars and asked them for their autograph. She then turned to her mother and said, 'One day some other young girl is going to make her way across this room and ask for my autograph.'

And she was right. As a teenager, she worked as a school teacher and married young, only to be divorced and remarried by the time she was nineteen to one Paul Mansfield. A couple of years later, by now with baby Jayne in tow, the family moved to Hollywood to pursue Jayne senior's lifelong dream of becoming a star.

Her husband only stayed with her for four months, and they divorced soon after, but Jayne remained and started working in a movie theatre as well as taking on part-time modelling work. In one of her early shoots, for General Electric, Jayne posed with a group of girls, but was cut out of the final image 'because she looked too sexy for 1954 viewers'.

However, Jayne Mansfield's appeal was spotted by a Hollywood publicity agent called Jim Byron, who booked her to pay a visit to newspaper offices to 'cheer up overworked reporters'. Can you imagine doing that these days?! Amazingly, Jayne's picture appeared in all the papers the next day and her career really took off. She appeared in several hit films, including *The Girl Can't Help It* and *Kiss Them For Me* opposite Cary Grant, but her life ended tragically when she was killed in a car accident at the age of thirty-four.

Jayne Mansfield was the ultimate scene-stealer: early on in her career she attended the launch of a Jane Russell film called *Underwater*, wearing nothing but a red bikini. Unsurprisingly, the media picked up on the way she'd stolen the limelight with headlines like *Jayne Out-Points Jane.*

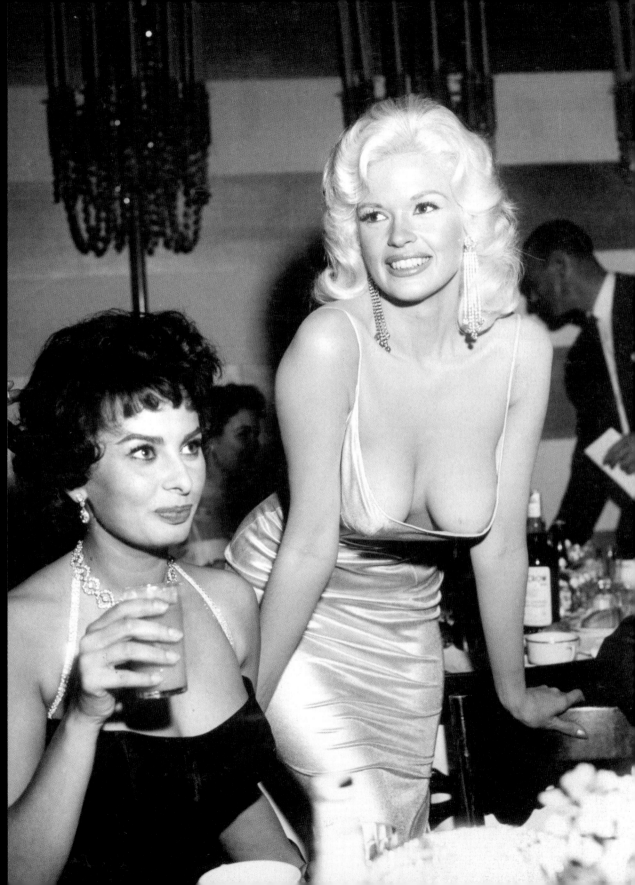

Later in her career, she went to see a Mae West performance and came away with one of the muscle men from Miss West's dance troupe, former Mr Universe Mickey Hargitay. Distressed that Mansfield had stolen the affections of one of her entourage, West summoned Hargitay to a press conference and ordered him to denounce his relationship with Jayne, but instead of reading the scripted statement, to West's horror, he simply said, 'Jayne and I are very much in love and we have seriously discussed marriage plans in the future.' Mansfield and Hargitay did marry and went on to have three children, living in her famous 'Pink Palace' on Hollywood's Sunset Boulevard until they divorced in 1964.

Jayne also stole the show at a 1957 party to welcome Sophia Loren to Hollywood, where the sultry Italian star was photographed seated at dinner next to her, transfixed by Mansfield's voluptuous bosom while Mansfield herself simply smiled adoringly at the camera – now that's a star!

Although Jayne Mansfield is often labelled a second-rate Marilyn Monroe, I think she had her own unique qualities. Yes, she was a peroxide blonde who played on her girlish charms and womanly silhouette, but she was an incredibly ambitious woman who had a definite sense of her own destiny. She was also renowned for being a very kind, gentle human being, and although she used to earn a fortune for her cabaret act in Las Vegas, she never became a diva and remained devoted to her family.

Cyd Charisse

Born in 1921, in Texas, Tula Ellice Finklea allegedly gained the nickname Cyd when her brother mispronounced 'sis'. She had ballet lessons from a young age and grew up wanting to be a dancer. Eventually her passion took her to Hollywood, where she starred alongside the likes of Gene Kelly in the 1952 classic *Singing in the Rain* and Fred Astaire in a series of big-screen musicals.

So renowned was she for her graceful, long, nimble limbs that in 1952, an insurance company accepted a five-million-dollar policy on her legs, beating the previous record holder, Betty Grable.

She is one of those women who simply loved dancing, and it showed in every performance she gave. She was born to dance: it was as if she couldn't stand still, and her legs simply had to move. For me, it's a joy to watch that kind of talent.

Betty Grable

The most famous picture of Betty Grable was taken in 1943 by Frank Powolny: she is wearing a white bathing suit, photographed from behind, but looking over her shoulder and smiling at the camera, and it was to provide salvation for millions of GIs fighting overseas during the Second World War. As one of the first pin-up girls, this iconic image of Grable was voted by *Life* magazine as one of the 100 photographs that changed the world, and was particularly inspirational to me when I was invited to pay a morale-boosting visit to British servicemen stationed in Bosnia in 1997.

Although she never actually travelled to visit troops overseas, Grable actively participated in the domestic war effort, appearing at camps across the USA and auctioning off her nylon stockings for thousands of dollars. She was dedicated to the American military and always tried to respond to her fan mail, which often amounted to 10,000 letters a week.

Born Elizabeth Ruth Grable in 1916, Betty, as she was known, was pushed into dancing at an early age by her mother. By the age of thirteen, she was working as a chorus girl for Fox Studios, but was fired when they discovered she was younger than the legal age for film work. Betty went on to work for all the major Hollywood studios, and eventually signed a lucrative contract with Fox, becoming their number-one box office star in the early 1940s.

Grable was renowned for her shapely legs, and insured them for one million dollars apiece with Lloyds of London, making them the most valuable pins in the world.

I adore the fact that Grable was such an iconic figure to all those young servicemen, and that a simple picture could keep hope alive for homesick men who might never come home. She symbolised a wholesome, sensual womanliness that was acceptable during the Second World War, and the very fact that she was celebrating femininity so those fighting on the front line could escape the harsh realities of war is something that should be recognised.

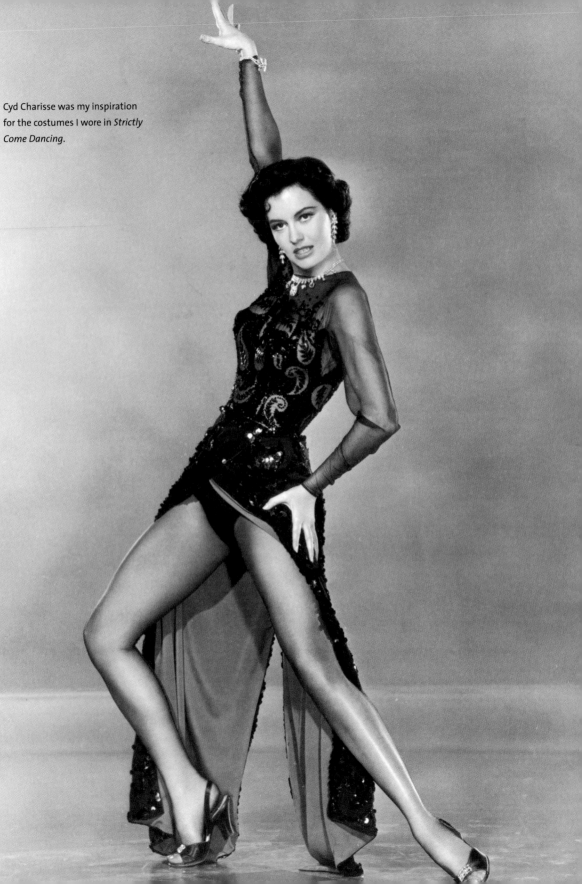

Cyd Charisse was my inspiration for the costumes I wore in *Strictly Come Dancing*.

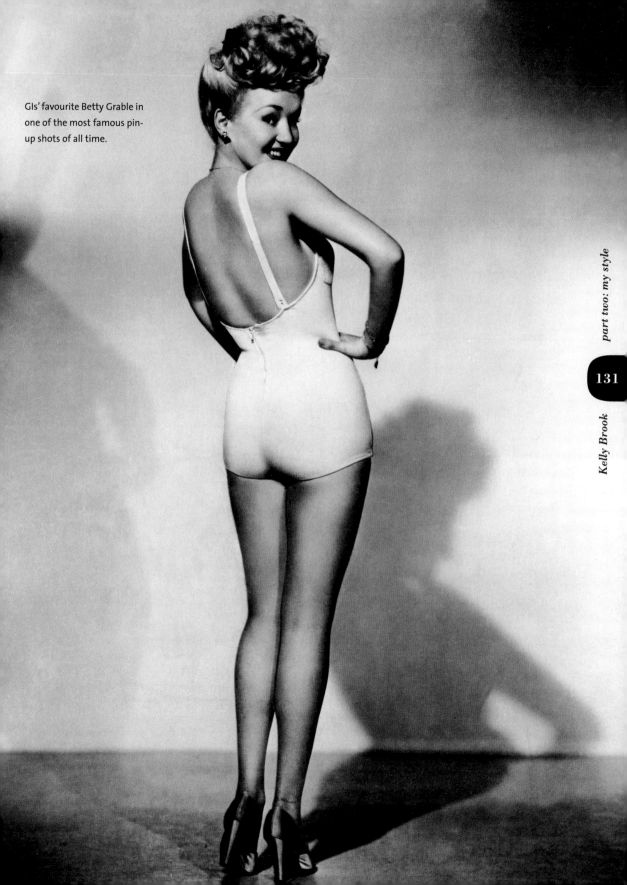

GIs' favourite Betty Grable in one of the most famous pin-up shots of all time.

Marilyn Monroe ordered handmade shoes from the Italian designer Salvatore Ferragamo, who always made one heel about one quarter of an inch lower than the other. Why? So Marilyn would walk with her trademark wiggle. I'm not suggesting you go to those lengths, though, as it's probably not very good for your joints to have one heel higher than the other.

Marilyn Monroe

Norma Jeane Baker was born in Los Angeles in June 1926. Her childhood was blighted by sexual abuse at the hands of a string of men, and in the absence of a father, her mother, Gladys Baker (née Monroe) struggled to support her daughter. It wasn't long before Norma Jeane moved into a series of foster homes and orphanages after her mother's unstable mental health meant she was institutionalised. It's hardly surprising that when Jim Dougherty, a twenty-one-year-old aircraft engineer, proposed to a sixteen-year-old Norma Jeane, she jumped at the chance to escape her unsettled life. Though their marriage lasted only four years, it was during this period that she bleached her hair and began working as a swimsuit model and posing for pin-up photos.

It wasn't long before Hollywood executives spotted the potential of the young model, and Twentieth Century Fox signed her to a six-month, $125-a-week contract, changing her name to Marilyn Monroe as part of the deal.

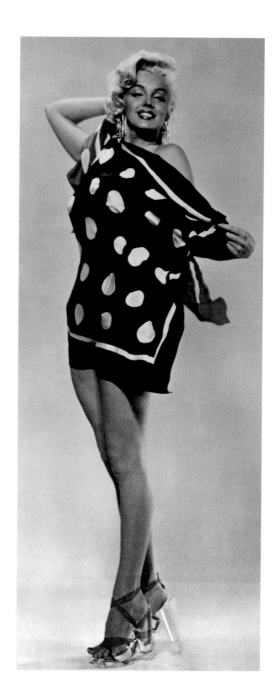

right: Marilyn Monroe remains a style icon to this day.

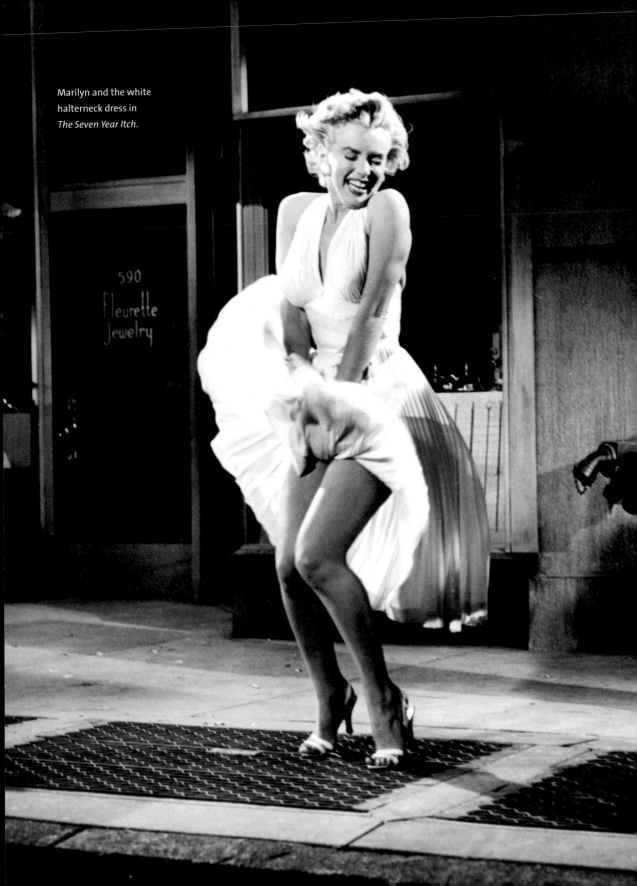

Marilyn and the white
halterneck dress in
The Seven Year Itch.

590
Fleurette
Jewelry

Marilyn Monroe had a warmth and charm you can't buy: it wasn't about her clothes or her bleached blonde hair, but about her fragile vulnerability combined with an incredible sensuality.

She was the ultimate girl-woman, with her childlike eyes and pouting mouth atop the body of a goddess. She spoke like a child, with the knowing allure of an experienced woman. To me, Marilyn was sunshine.

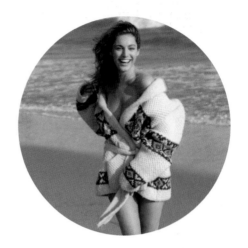

I love the fact that Marilyn's body was by no means perfect: in today's terms she was probably a voluptuous size 16, with generous thighs and hips. But she was comfortable with her shape and happy to be photographed in revealing sheer dresses and skimpy bikinis. It was that grown-up confidence, combined with a childlike need to be loved that made her so appealing.

She was a style icon, but there are probably only a couple of her outfits that are truly memorable: the sunray-pleated white halterneck dress she wore over the subway grating in *The Seven Year Itch* with her skirt flying high around her thighs. And then the sparkling column that was so tight she was sewn into it to sing 'Happy Birthday, Mr President' to John F. Kennedy. Other than that, she is remembered more for the 'essence of Marilyn': the kooky voice, the bleached white hair, the pale skin combined with black eyeliner and scarlet lips. She created her own identity, which gave her a memorable style.

A make-up artist I work with on a regular basis, Kim Goodwin, has been collecting prints of Marilyn for a number of years, and owns some beautiful photographs of her wearing a chunky intarsia-knit fawn sweater on the beach. She looks so playful and carefree in those pictures and I've always loved them, so Kim surprised me one day with a replica sweater he'd made. We went out and did some photographs of me in a similar style, and he gave them to me as a gift.

Kim also gave me two framed portraits by André de Diene, one of Marilyn's early boyfriends, and I have two stunning nude prints of her on the wall at my house. She's a constant source of inspiration, and despite the tragedy that engulfed and ended her life at just thirty-six, she remains a style icon for many women to this day.

above: Me in the replica sweater that Kim Goodwin had made to echo the one Marilyn wore in the famous shots by George Barris.

Veronica Lake

On 14 November 1919, Constance Frances Marie Ockelman was born in Brooklyn, New York, and by the age of eight she'd made her stage debut in a school production of *Poor Little Rich Girl*. After losing her father in an oil ship accident when she was just twelve, Constance's mother remarried and she adopted her stepfather's name, Keane. The family moved to Canada, back to New York and then to Florida, and when Constance was nineteen, she won the Miss Florida beauty pageant, but was later disqualified and stripped of her title because she'd misled the judges about her age.

That same year, she moved to Hollywood with her mother and stepfather and enrolled at the Bliss Hayden School of Acting, securing small parts in a number of movies. One day during filming her fine blonde hair fell over her eyes, and the director insisted the scene be shot like that. Her famous peek-a-boo style was born, but it wasn't until 1941 that she gained her stage name, when Paramount producer Arthur Hornblow Jr declared, 'I believe that when people look into those navy-blue eyes of yours, they'll see a calm coolness – the calm of a lake – and your features, Connie, are classic features. And when I think of classic features, I think Veronica.'

right: Veronica Lake's alluring hairstyle was hugely influential.

Veronica Lake's influence on the hairstyles of a generation was such that government officials had to beg her to stop wearing her hair long for the duration of the Second World War, because women working in munitions plants were catching their long hair in machines.

I love the way her hair became her trademark; its artful style made her look incredibly alluring, as if she were peeping out from behind a silk curtain. If I'm attending a glamorous red-carpet event, I often ask my hair stylist to put my hair in big rollers and recreate the seductive Veronica Lake look.

The other thing we can all learn from her is that sometimes we find a look that we weren't planning on – in her case, her hair falling over her eyes – but as soon as we see it, we know it works. In that case, go for it. So if you see something in the mirror that looks just right for you, don't carry on aiming for the style you'd originally planned.

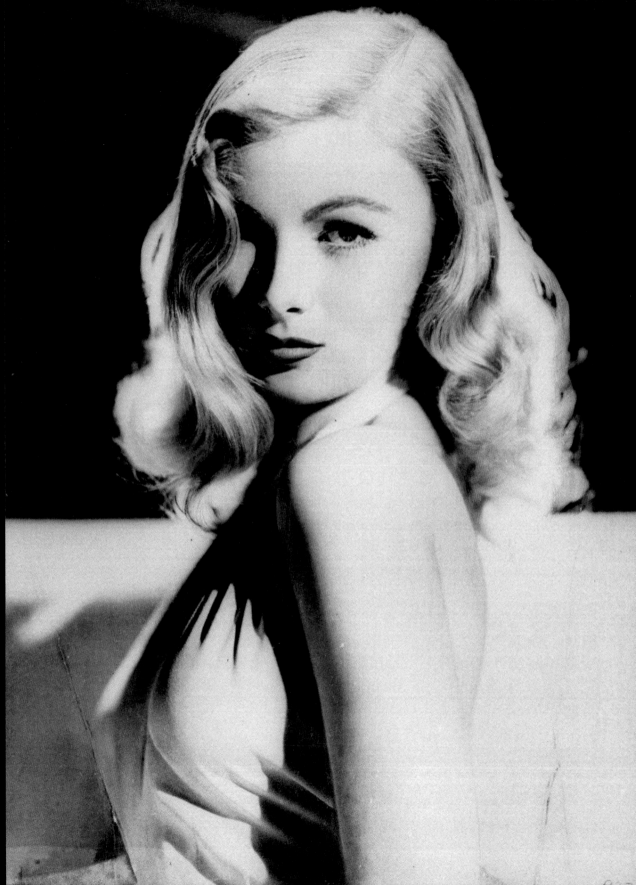

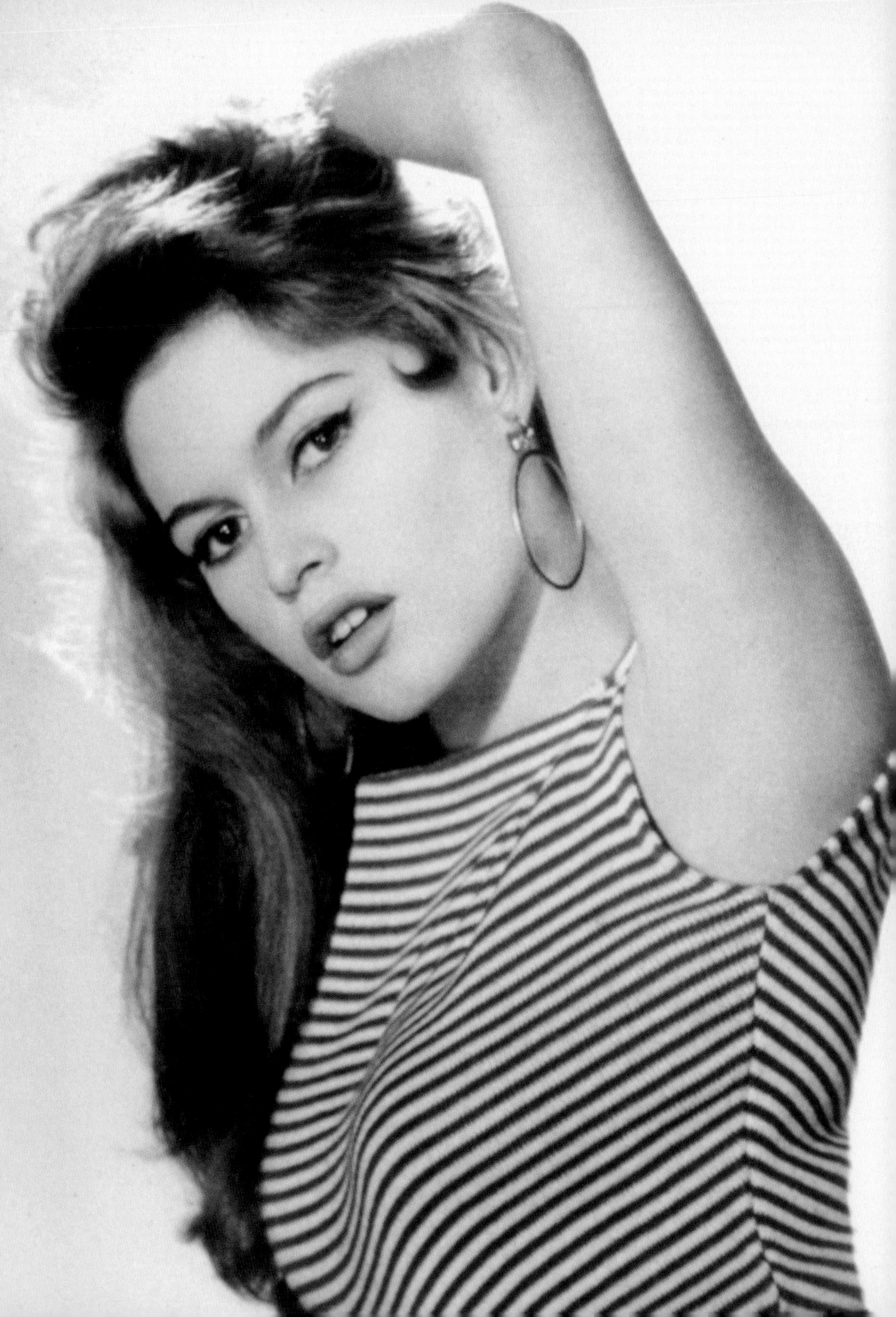

Brigitte Bardot

The same year Sophia Loren was born in Rome, Anne-Marie Mucel and industrialist Charles Bardot celebrated the arrival of their daughter, Camille, in Paris. They raised her in a strict religious, conservative family environment, with her mother encouraging her to study music and dance from an early age. However, as she entered her teens, blossoming into a beautiful young woman, their daughter rebelled.

Brigitte Bardot began her career as a teenage model, and appeared on her first magazine cover – *Elle* – when she was only fourteen. She had a Lolita quality that entranced the film director Roger Vadim, and the pair soon became romantically involved. The couple eventually announced they were to marry, but Bardot's parents refused point blank to endorse the wedding, allegedly leaving the teenage beauty suicidal. However, when she turned eighteen, she went ahead and married her lover anyway, only to find herself a divorcee five years later.

Though their marriage was short-lived, Vadim was highly instrumental in launching Bardot's career and turning her into a movie starlet. She was lionised as a French icon, and became the unofficial face and body of the Cote d'Azur and the Cannes Film Festival, attracting a new, young glamorous crowd to the south of France.

left: Brigitte Bardot in the sort of Gallic top I also love to wear.

Though she was fêted as the sex goddess of the decade in 1950s Europe, her highly erotic film presence was deemed too controversial for American audiences. She starred alongside Kirk Douglas in one US production, *Un Acte d'Amour*, but Bardot never really got her big break into Hollywood, and stepped away from showbusiness when she turned forty, choosing instead to become a political campaigner and animal rights activist.

I love the way that, as a young woman, Brigitte Bardot played on her coquettish, naïve charm. She was the ultimate sex kitten with her tousled, just-out-of-bed hair and sensual, pale pout. Her heavy eyeliner only served to emphasise her come-hither eyes, and she had great fun flirting with the world.

In contrast to the polished presentation of Sophia Loren and the blatant sexual teasing of Bettie Page, Brigitte Bardot was the insouciant plaything. She had a casual charm that felt like she hadn't tried. She made capri pants, ballet pumps and Gallic tops her trademark, but it wasn't like she'd gone out to create a signature style; instead it was a case of 'that's just what I like to wear'.

In our modern world, where images are carefully crafted by stylists and PR gurus, I love the Bardot take-me-or-leave-me attitude. Like so many of my idols, I think she shows women how important it is to feel relaxed and comfortable in what we wear. That's how we can ensure we look our best, even if the clothes aren't actually that special in themselves.

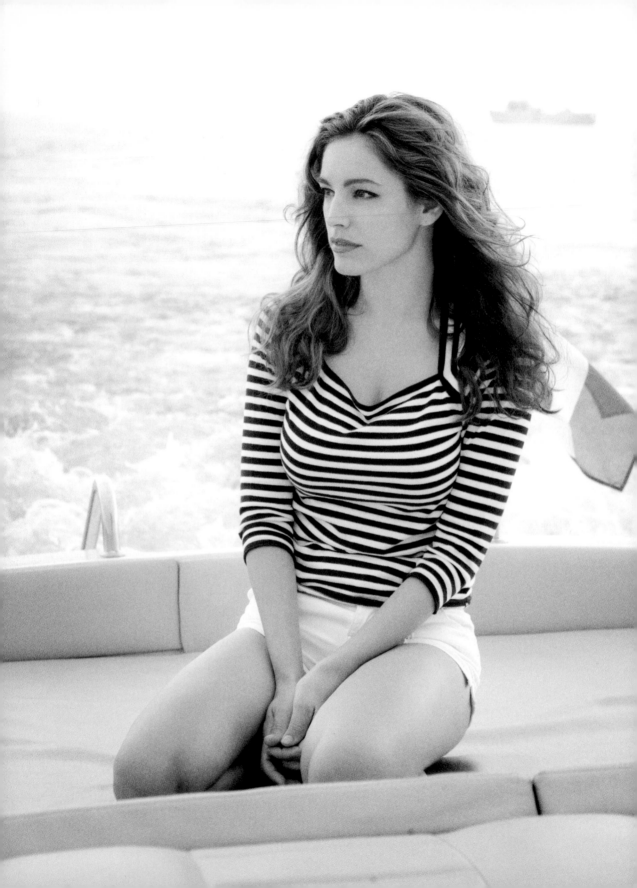

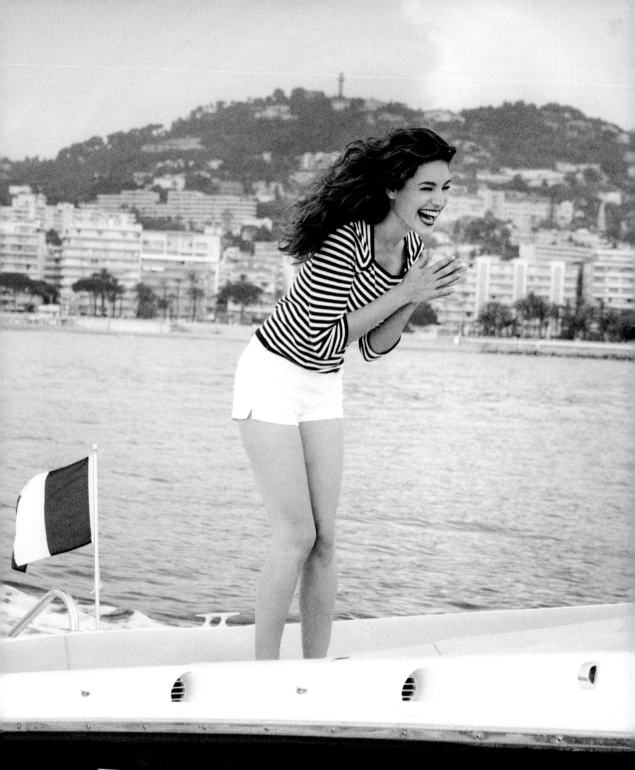

pin-up artists ⑫

Of course, it's not always the pin-ups themselves who create their inspirational images, sometimes it is artists, photographers and stylists. The people I have chosen in this chapter are those who have created some of the most stunning images of women. If you look at their work, you will find so many ideas to help you create your own style – I know I have. The key thing is not simply to look at current fashion magazines, but to take your inspiration from wherever you find it.

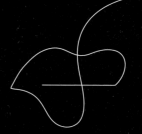

Alberto Vargas

Born in Peru in 1896, the son of a photographer, Alberto Vargas studied art and photography in Europe before moving to New York at the age of twenty. Though he had intended to go home to Peru, he was entranced by the self-confidence of young American women and decided to remain in the US, where he began working as an artist for the Ziegfeld Follies on Broadway, as well as various Hollywood studios, where he painted stars such as Barbara Stanwyck, Marlene Dietrich and Shirley Temple. But it wasn't until the early 1940s, when he began creating watercolour and airbrush pin-ups for *Esquire* magazine, that he really came to public prominence.

So popular were these 'cheesecake' images of wholesome yet sexy all-American girls that they were used to adorn military aircraft during the Second World War, and 'Varga girls' became the generic label for semi-nude, American pin-ups. His eponymous works were the symbol of American life and served as a beacon of hope for the young servicemen fighting for their country – one day, they dreamed, they would go home to a country where these apple-pie beauties were plentiful.

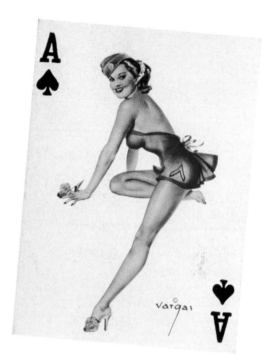

Above: 'Varga girls' were all the rage in the 1940s.

He later went on to work for *Playboy* magazine, creating ever more naked portraits of beautiful women and establishing himself as the finest artist of the pin-up genre.

I am constantly enthralled by Vargas, whose talent for portraying female sexuality on canvas is unmatched in my opinion. Even in his later years, in the Seventies, when *Playboy* ordered him to start showing pubic hair – against his own better judgement – he still gave his pin-ups a dignity and femininity that others couldn't have achieved.

When I am working on ideas for my calendar or for a swimwear shoot, I regularly use his work as a reference point: his eye for a flattering yet provocative pose was incredible, and I'll often look to his portraits as inspiration when I'm modelling.

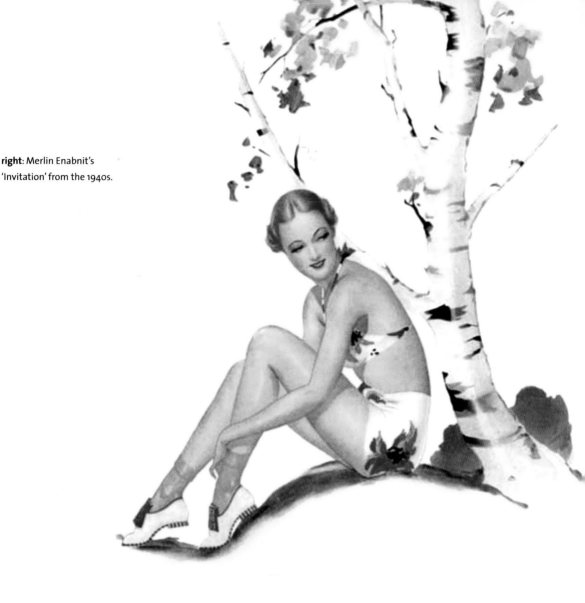

right: Merlin Enabnit's
'Invitation' from the 1940s.

Merlin Enabnit

Merlin Enabnit was born in Des Moines, Iowa, in 1903 and began sketching on wrapping paper in his father's grocery store when he was still a young boy. As a professional artist, he painted in various mediums and covered an array of subject matter, from commercial packaging to landscapes and pin-up girls.

His work was incredibly diverse, with some illustrations in gentle watercolours and others in bolder primary colours, but there is one constant: I love the way he portrays women as curvaceous beauties with a sense of fun; they're always feminine and flirty, which is the essence of the perfect pin-up.

David Wright

Most of the famous pin-up artists were American, but the British illustrator David Wright managed to make a name for himself with his own unique style. After leaving school at thirteen, he went to work for his uncle, who was a newsprint artist. Wright soon learned the technique of figurative art and began to take commissions for fashion illustrations from the women's weekly magazines.

In 1941, at the age of twenty-nine, he got his big break, and was commissioned to produce a series of images of glamorous women, known as 'lovelies', for the *Sketch*. His softly coloured illustrations featured ladies in sheer negligées, or in various states of undress, many of which were modelled on his wife, Esme. During the Second World War, he was a driving instructor for the armed forces in Abersoch, Wales, where he worked on his illustrations during his spare time. Wright quickly became one of the most popular pin-up artists in Britain during the Second World War, and his work was considered a morale booster for those serving in the armed forces. Wright produced a total of 169 prints and one cover for the *Sketch* over a period of ten years.

In the 1950s, he began to work for *Men Only* magazine, and also created the Carol Day cartoon strip for the *Daily Mail*, which mirrored the soap opera cartoon style that was also appearing in the US at the time.

For me, Wright's work has a lightness of touch that contrasts with the work of his American counterparts. Rather than using an airbrush to colour his work, he tended to use watercolours, which gives the illustrations a softer feel. I think he captures the essence of feminine allure beautifully, with seductive poses, tantalising lingerie and pretty, often seemingly demure, women.

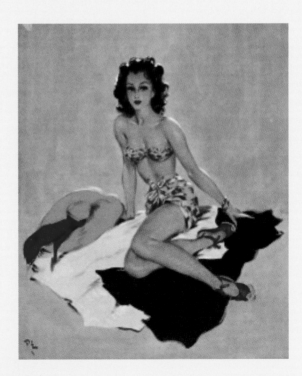

right: 'Tan Talizing', David Wright's soft colours and seductive poses are so appealing.

the foundations of style

Underwear is one of the most important elements of a woman's wardrobe. It's all too easy to pretend it doesn't matter because it's not on show, and instead spend your hard-earned cash on shoes, bags, dresses and jewels, but just like a building – you see, I did learn something from my scaffolder father! – if you get the foundations wrong, the whole structure will come tumbling down around you. If you start from the inside out when creating your look you'll find you dress with much more confidence – after all, what's the point in decorating a house when the walls are cracked and there's subsidence?

In fact, even before you get to the first layer of your clothes, you must remember that it is your skin that comes into contact with what you are wearing. So the first thing to do is ensure that your skin is in the best condition possible. I do this by regularly using body scrubs and body oils so I am ready to slip on the first layer of wrapping. I don't weigh myself regularly, and I honestly believe that if the man you love says you look gorgeous, then you shouldn't beat yourself up over a few pounds. When I first started modelling, agents would tell me I was too short or too curvy, and would suggest I lose some weight. Thankfully I had the confidence to ignore them, because I was healthy and content with my shape. I'm not perfect, by any means, but I am me and I am happy with what nature has given me. For all of us, our body shapes can help or hinder us, depending on what we want to do; there is no such thing as the right shape.

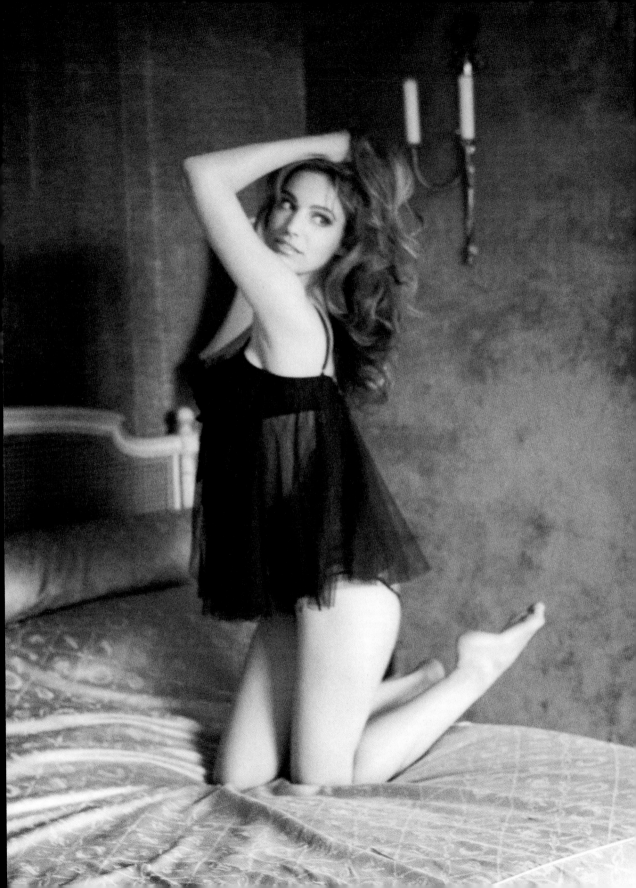

I look after my body, but I'm not obsessive about it, because you have to have a life: I enjoy food and I'm not a gym bunny. I like to have sugar in my tea, and a chocolate chip cookie to dunk in it, too, but I don't feel guilty about indulging. I just make sure I also eat plenty of healthy foods, so I get enough fruit and veg and all the right nutrients. Everything in moderation, I say, and if you follow that rule you can walk around with a smile on your face.

I absolutely adore beautiful lingerie, but it's important to remember that, as well as the sexy pieces you have for the bedroom, you need a complete underwear wardrobe that works with your everyday clothes and eveningwear, too. So, just like you have stiletto-heeled strappy sandals to wear with your cocktail dresses, you'll need the right underwear to match. When you pop on your trainers and workout gear, it's important to wear the right bra to give you support while you exercise, and though a pink, frilled lacy number might be perfect for a flirty seduction, it simply won't work under a smooth, stretchy T-shirt.

But before we look at what I consider to be the perfect capsule lingerie wardrobe, the most important thing to do first is to get measured. I know from bitter experience what it's like to wear the wrong size bra – when I first started modelling, so many of the styles I liked weren't available in my cup size, so I'd end up squeezing myself into something that was too small. Not only was it uncomfortable, it looked ridiculous.

without fou
there can b

Today, it's estimated that about 70 per cent of British women wear the wrong bra size – you can often tell, even when women are walking down the street, because their bra is clearly visible riding up their back or they're oozing over the top of the cups – so I reckon it's worth swallowing your pride and making an appointment for a professional fitting. Most department stores and lingerie boutiques offer a complementary measuring service, and I strongly recommend taking them up on it. It's all too easy to keep buying the same bra size for years, forgetting that our body shape changes. Just because you can still do it up, it doesn't necessarily mean the size you wore ten years ago is the right size for you now. Many women's bra sizes vary throughout their monthly cycle – it's not uncommon to go up a whole size during menstruation, and continuing to wear your normal bra size might lead to discomfort, especially if you suffer from tender tissue at this time of the month – so it's worth being measured at different stages in case you need to go up a cup size for a few days each month.

ndation

e no fashion

Christian Dior

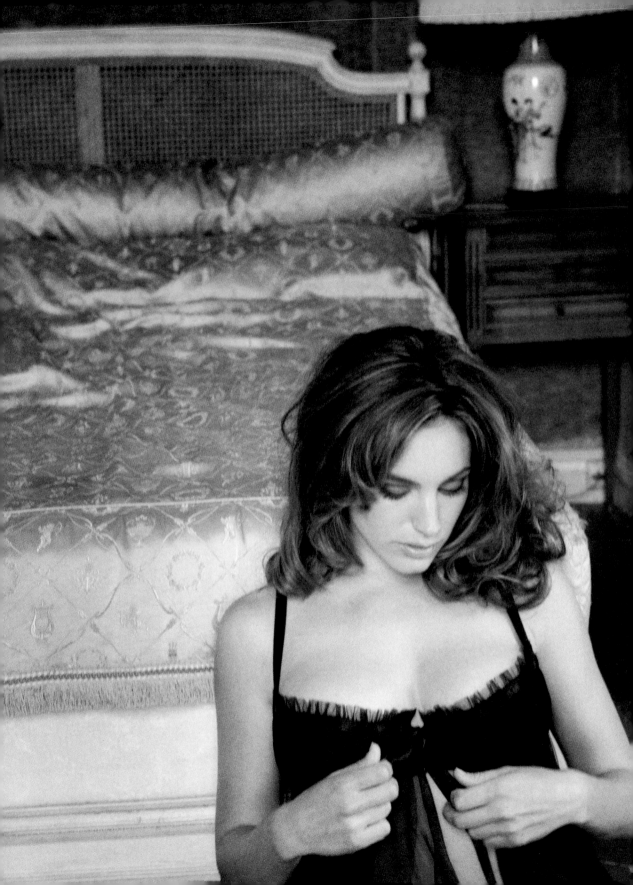

Many women don't fully understand the methodology of bra sizing and just add a familiar size to their basket without even trying it on; when they put on a correctly fitting bra, it can be a life-changing experience.

The most common mistake women make is wearing a bra that's too big around the torso, with a cup size that's too small. For example, wearing a 36B when they are, in fact, a 34D. While you may be able scoop your breasts into the cups and do up the back, an ill-fitting bra can damage your posture, cause unsightly lumps and bumps and even cut into sensitive tissue.

So, how can you tell if you are wearing the wrong size bra? If you can answer 'yes' to any of the following it's probably time to get yourself measured:

- The fastening band rides up my back and sits higher at the back than the front
- The fastening band feels tight or leaves a red mark around my torso
- My breasts bulge over the sides of the cups
- The underwires leave red marks on my breasts
- The centre-front of the bra doesn't sit flat between my breasts
- The underwires ride up over my breasts and I have to adjust them throughout the day
- My bra straps dig into my shoulders, leaving red marks
- The bra cups are crinkly or sag on my breasts

I promise you, if you've been wearing the wrong size bra, the moment you put on one that fits you'll walk taller, your breasts will look better and you'll feel so much more comfortable. Not only that, it does wonders for a girl's confidence.

Once you've been measured, it's important to try on bras before you buy them: just as with clothes, different manufacturers and different styles will vary the fitting, so a 34B in one brand won't necessarily be the same as a 34B in another. You know your foot size, but you'd always try on shoes before buying them, wouldn't you? So, why do any different with bras? Your body will thank you in the long run.

There are so many different underwear styles out there, and it's important to know what your options are before you start shopping. Once you know what different terms mean, you'll be a better-informed consumer, so here's my guide to lingerie vocabulary.

Baby doll

This sexy boudoir garment is not strictly lingerie, as I can't think of anything you could feasibly wear it under. However, the baby doll definitely has its place in a girl's trousseau. Usually empire line, and made from sheer tulle or chiffon, it's a thigh-skimming number with matching panties, and is incredibly seductive and flirty.

Balconette bra

A very pretty, feminine bra shape usually with quarter or half cups, cut horizontally across the bust line to create uplift, with the help of underwiring and sometimes under-breast padding. Balconette bras lift and separate the breasts, rather than pushing them together, and usually have wide-set straps, so the effect is one of your breasts being 'served' on a balcony.

Bandeau bra

A strapless style, usually smooth and made from stretchy fabric, like a cropped boob tube. Only suitable for smaller-busted women.

Boyshorts

Fitted briefs, usually cut fairly low on the midiff and horizontally across the top of the thigh, just below the buttock line. Cute and sexy on younger women, but not always flattering on a more mature body.

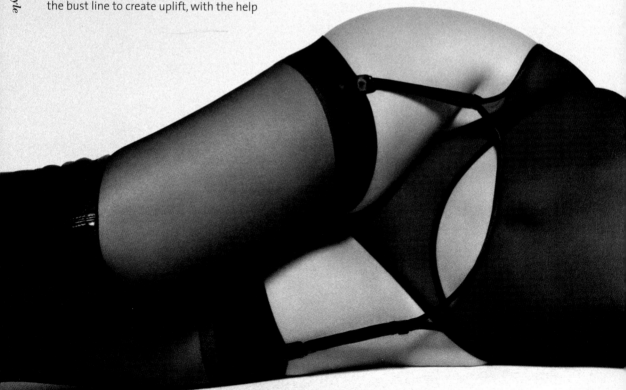

Brazilian-back briefs

These high-cut briefs cover more of your bottom than a thong, but not as much as a traditional brief – not one to wear if you're worried about VPL!

Bustier

Usually strapless, with underwired cups, this is a bra extended into a bodice-shape, usually done up at the rear with a series of hook-and-eye fastenings. They're often stiffened using 'boning' – in the old days this was literally strips of whalebone, but now thankfully it's usually plastic – and are particularly popular under evening dresses and bridal gowns.

Camisole

A spaghetti-strapped body-skimming waist-length top, sometimes incorporating 'soft' bra cups, traditionally made from a drapable fabric like silk crêpe de Chine or lightweight satin. Modern camisoles are often made from cotton blended with elastane for a streamlined shape, and sometimes they have an in-built soft bra inside, so they can be worn as a top in their own right.

One of my favourite lingerie shots, by Rankin.

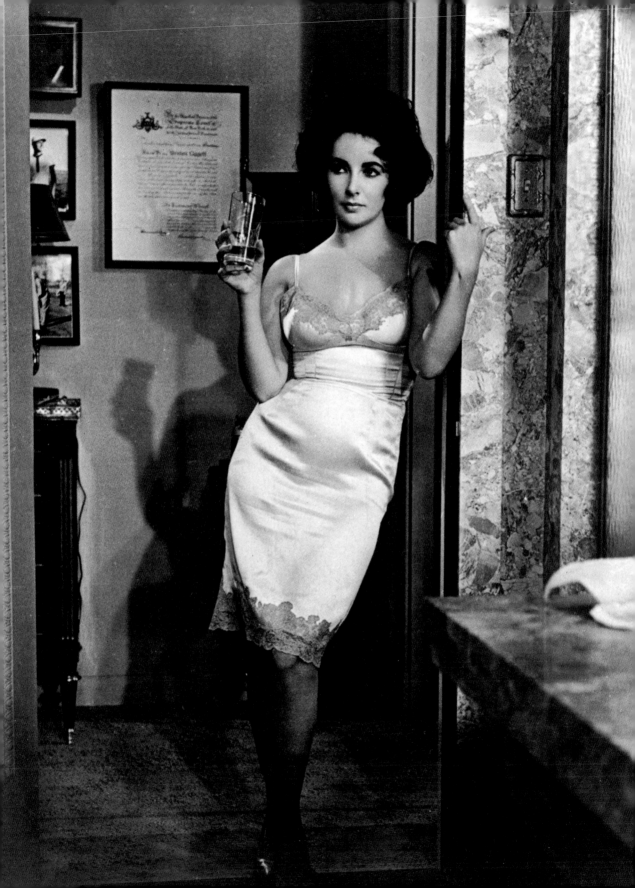

Chicken fillets

Not strictly underwear, but definitely part of many women's top drawer. These fleshy little parcels are literally shaped like chicken fillets, and are inserted into a bra to add a little 'oomph' where Mother Nature hasn't done it herself. Definitely preferable to stuffing loo roll into your bra, chicken fillets have endowed millions of smaller-busted women with a cleavage for the first time in their lives.

Control briefs (or shorts)

Once upon a time only mature ladies would wear control underwear, but nowadays a host of Hollywood stars have confessed to controlling the bulge with specialist briefs. They might not be the sexiest undies around, but if you're wearing a fitted or body-skimming outfit, they can give you a streamlined shape when nature hasn't blessed you with one.

Convertible bra

Just what it says on the packet! A convertible bra offers a variety of permutations to wear under different garments, e.g., halterneck, cross-back, strapless, one shoulder, backless, etc. Personally I think they're a bit of a sales gimmick, but if you can find one that works for you, who am I to criticise?

left: Elizabeth Taylor displays the classic slip – timelessly glamorous.

Corset

A corset is a very fitted, structured garment, usually boned and laced at the front or rear to create an hourglass silhouette. Though inspired by traditional Victorian and Edwardian styles, modern-day corsets are rarely tightened to the extremes they were then, and are often made from comfortable stretchy fabrics. Some corsets have straps while others are strapless, and they also vary in length – some sit at the waist, others below the hipline – and some feature a structured cup while others merely squeeze the breasts upwards to create a rounded mound above the corsetline. Many women choose to wear corsets as outerwear, influenced by stars such as Madonna – remember her fabulous Jean Paul Gaultier cone-cupped style? – and designers such as Vivienne Westwood.

French knickers

A loose, long brief, like elasticated shorts, usually made from exotic fabrics such as satin or lace.

Full slip

What can I say? Think Elizabeth Taylor in *Cat on a Hot Tin Roof* and you'll appreciate the allure of a body-skimming silk, lace-trimmed slip. Some think they're old-fashioned, but I think they can be incredibly glamorous and a great alternative to obviously sexy underwear when you want to be subtly feminine.

G-string

Pretty much the skimpiest item of lingerie there is, the G-string is a tiny triangle of fabric at the front, joined at the sides and underneath by elastic, ribbon, or even a string of pearls for the truly daring!

Garter

An elasticated band, usually trimmed with ribbons and lace, and traditionally worn around the thigh to help keep stockings in place. They're largely superfluous in today's wardrobes, when elastane, often known by the brand name Lycra®, keeps hosiery up, but they're still popular with brides. I rather like the idea of wearing a garter with stockings – they're a piece of frivolity and can be fun when you're seducing a lover.

Half-slip

A skirt-style slip worn to avoid static beneath unlined skirts or dresses, or to avoid a garment appearing see-through. They used to be a wardrobe staple in my grandmother's day, but they're not so common now. However, like a full slip, if you wear a tactile style in soft lace-trimmed silk, it can add a certain edge to undressing in front of your lover.

Hipster briefs (or hip-huggers)

Often described as low-rise briefs, these are perfect for wearing under low-cut jeans or trousers to avoid showing your knickers to the rest of the world. I know it's trendy among teenagers to show a glimpse of polyester thong in your builders' bum, but I think it's incredibly unattractive. Much better to go for a hipster brief that sits below the waistline of your jeans.

opposite: Suspender belts always add sex appeal.

Padded bras

Many different bra shapes can be padded to give a little extra boost to the bustline. Some are padded under the bust, to enhance uplift; some are padded at the side to push the breasts up and together, giving optimum cleavage; some are padded underneath and at the side – think the Wonderbra and you'll know the results this achieves – and some even have removable pads, often known as 'cookies', so that you have the option of wearing them or not, depending how much va va voom you're after on a particular day.

Plunge bra

A plunge bra usually has a very low centre-point, with angled-cups to wear with V necklines, and they're sometimes padded to create cleavage.

Push-up bra

Often padded underneath the breasts, the push-up bra is designed to maximise uplift, separating the breasts to create a defined rounded shape.

Soft-cup bra

This refers to any bra that doesn't feature underwiring. A soft-cup bra can come in a number of shapes and styles, but is usually better for smaller-busted women who don't need the support of a more structured bra.

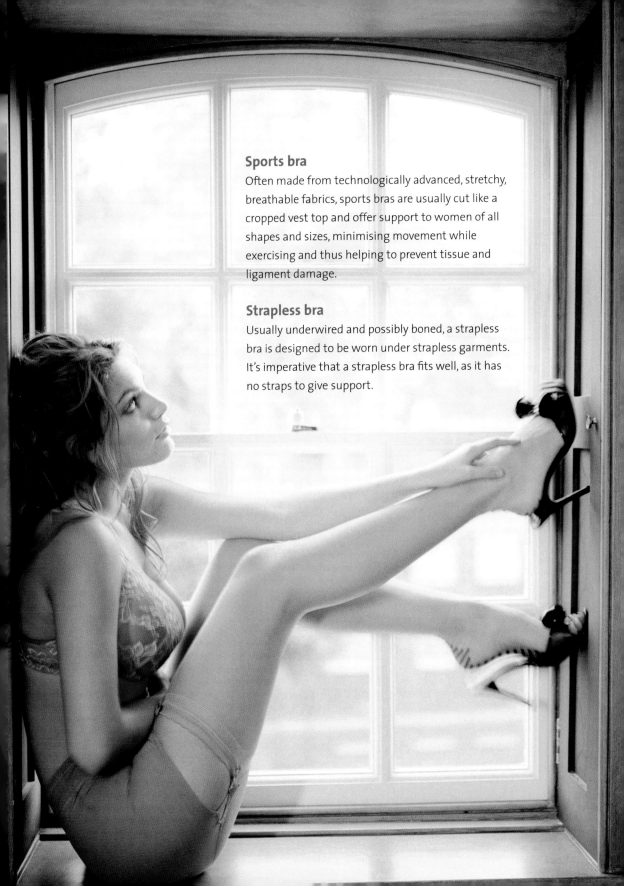

Sports bra

Often made from technologically advanced, stretchy, breathable fabrics, sports bras are usually cut like a cropped vest top and offer support to women of all shapes and sizes, minimising movement while exercising and thus helping to prevent tissue and ligament damage.

Strapless bra

Usually underwired and possibly boned, a strapless bra is designed to be worn under strapless garments. It's imperative that a strapless bra fits well, as it has no straps to give support.

"I've yet to find the man who doesn't adore stockings and suspenders"

String bikini

Briefs with a narrow side, often simply a piece of elastic or ribbon, and usually with a high-cut leg. They generally have medium bottom coverage.

Suspender belt

Usually made to match a bra and panty set, the suspender belt is a rather old-fashioned but very glamorous garment, with four stretchy suspenders clipped on to your stocking tops. Though considered ridiculously impractical by most modern women, I've yet to find the man who doesn't adore stockings and suspenders. I think they add a certain *frisson* if you wear them on a date, and your man will definitely love watching you peel it off later – if, of course, he gets that far!

T-shirt bra

A modern term, coined to describe a smooth, usually flesh-toned – although they do come in white, black and other neutrals, too – bra that can be worn under stretchy or fitted garments to give shape and support without unsightly lines. They often take advantage of manufacturing technology, and frequently have seamless, heat-moulded cups to ensure breast-shaping without unsightly seams.

Tap pants

Fitted shorts that give full coverage but have a flirty feel to them. Think of the styles worn by tap dancers in the 1930s – usually in lace-trimmed satin – and you'll have an idea what these are like.

Teddy

First worn in the 1920s, teddies enjoyed their heyday in the 1970s and early 1980s. Designed like a camisole with briefs or shorts attached, they're not always the most comfortable of garments and can be ungainly if you have to visit the bathroom or want to do a seductive striptease for your lover. For me, they're a bit like the bodysuits Donna Karan invented: a great idea, but not very practical.

Thong

In America, thongs are what we in England call flip-flops, i.e., simple beach sandals with a toe-post. However, thongs in the lingerie lexicon are briefs cut small at the back so they leave the buttocks bared. NB. A thong is usually more substantial than a G-string.

Waspie

This waist-cinching garment has its origins in the 1950s and is like a boned belt that you wear with a bra and briefs to give waist definition. They can be made from anything – lace, satin, whatever – and usually fasten with hooks and eyes, laces, zippers or snap-fasteners. They're a much sexier alternative to control underwear, but if you're wearing something fitted, a waspie will show through.

opposite: Plunge bras are great to wear with v necklines.

Kelly's lingerie wardrobe

14

On a day-to-day basis, I believe the most important concern for any woman's lingerie is comfort. Yes, I like my underwear to look nice, but if it doesn't feel good, then no amount of expensive lace is going to make it up to me. Because of my size, I never go without a bra – unless I'm wearing an evening dress with in-built support – and I recommend that even smaller-busted women shouldn't either.

It's important that a woman should have a good range of items of lingerie to reflect their range of activities. What follows is a list of some of the key items in my underwear wardrobe and when I'll wear them, which I hope will give you an idea of the sorts of things you might think about.

When I'm at home, shopping or just pottering about with friends, I'd suggest going for a simple, smooth T-shirt bra in a neutral flesh tone, which offers good support and creates a good line under my clothes. I like natural fibres, where possible, and usually wear a full-cup shape so it's supportive.

I don't believe you need to be obsessive about matching bras and knickers: sometimes I'll wear a flesh-toned bra under a white shirt, with a brightly coloured mesh thong by Cosabella, one of my favourite everyday staples. They come in a rainbow of different shades and are really comfortable. I like thongs for everyday as I can't bear VPL: one of my style rules is that I don't think you should ever see underwear beneath clothing.

If you're wearing a loose shirt you can get away with something more decorative underneath; I like to wear bras made from feminine fabrics or perhaps embroidered or trimmed with bows. My pet hate though is cheap, itchy lace.

Because delicate, expensive lingerie needs extra care when washing, I'd recommend sticking to good-quality basics most of the time: cotton briefs and simple bras that can be washed on a low temperature in the machine. It's important to use a lingerie bag to protect them from snagging, and make sure you wash them on a really low temperature and low spin speed: so many bras get ruined because they're washed too hot, or spun so fast the underwires get bent. Use a gentle detergent specifically made for delicates, too, even if you're washing your everyday undies.

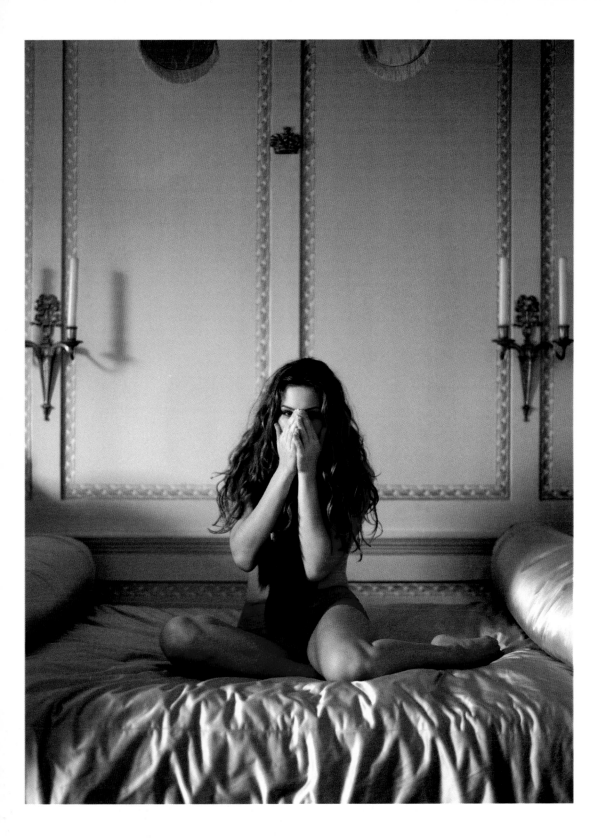

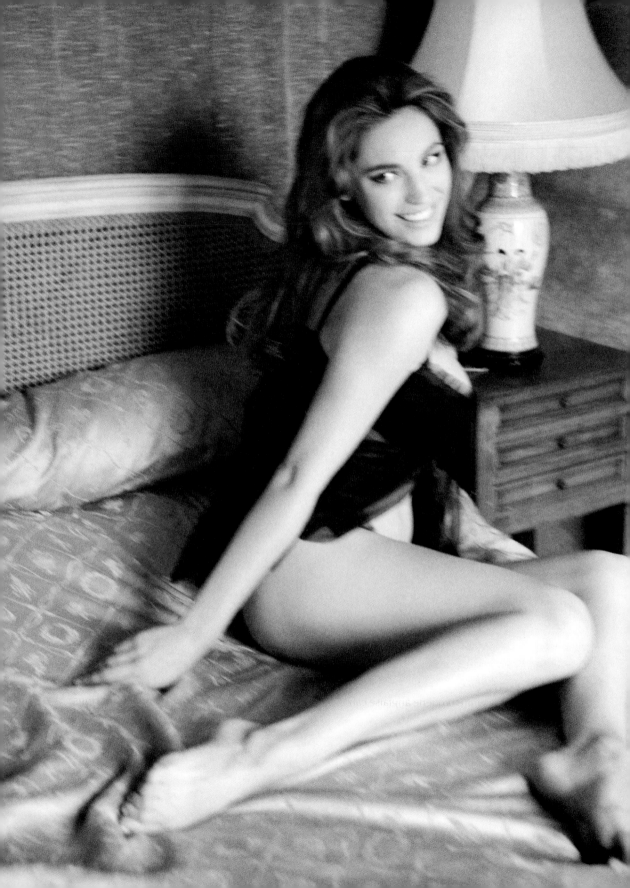

When it comes to bras, I wear different styles according to the clothes I'm wearing: sometimes a balconette style works best, while at other times a plunge bra enhancing my cleavage is better. Be flexible according to your circumstances.

If you're dressing up, I think it's worth really going for it with some fabulous underwear, which I absolutely adore. I have a great selection of different styles and fabrics, depending on what I'm wearing and what I'm in the mood for. For example, I love big knickers – I think they're incredibly sexy, especially frilly ones. I have a few pairs of wonderful frivolous frilly knickers from Agent Provocateur. I also enjoy trimmings such as bows: there's a British brand called Damaris which does fabulous panties with big silk bows and a peephole at the back; they're really beautiful.

Good quality silk, satins and lace are definitely important when it comes to that crucial feel-good factor. I enjoy having tactile fabrics next to my skin, and I think men love to touch soft, sensual fabrics when they are with a woman. Don't always go for the same coloured underwear, too: it's amazing how wearing a different colour can reflect or even change your mood. Red and black are definitely good for turning up the heat in sexual terms, whereas pretty pastel colours feel more demure, flirty and playful. Don't fall into the trap of thinking lingerie is only sexy if it's made from bright red lace, though: pretty white broderie anglaise can be just as alluring.

left: Feeling comfortable in what you wear can help bring a smile to your face.

I also have a soft spot for animal prints: and having fought hard to keep the leopard-spot bra and knickers in my lingerie collection for New Look, it turned out to be one of the range's bestsellers. There's something about animal prints that's really sensual: they can turn even the most timid temptress into a sexy seductress.

Stockings and suspenders are simply not practical on a day-to-day basis, but I love wearing them. If you're out on a hot date, wearing a pencil skirt and heels, you can't beat a suspender belt: just knowing you're wearing one makes you feel sexy, which in turn makes you behave differently.

For everyday, I wear good quality tights by Wolford or Fogal, either plain matte opaque ones or very sheer matte ones – I don't like shiny legs! I also love flesh-coloured fishnets, which go with almost anything, are surprisingly flattering and have a retro-glamour about them. It's definitely worth investing in good quality hosiery. It may seem an extravagance, but if you look after them – I always wear cotton gloves when I'm putting on stockings or tights – they last much longer than cheap brands and end up costing you less per wear than an inexpensive pair. I'm not from the label-loving, spend-more-every-time school of shopping, but I do think that buying cheap hosiery is a false economy.

At least nowadays there is a good range of bras on the market for people like me, but it wasn't always that way. Back in October 1998, on the back of all the lingerie shoots I'd been doing, I was signed as the Triumph girl, fronting – quite literally – an ad campaign promoting a new collection of bras for what they called the fuller-figured woman. The range was called Flaunt, and the idea was to use massive billboards across the country to flaunt their new range of larger cup size bras.

The company had undertaken extensive research and found that 10 per cent of bra sales in the UK were a DD-cup and above, with eighteen- to twenty-five-year-olds being the largest growing – excuse the pun! – group. Triumph wanted to tap into this market and had booked me to promote the range they planned to do it with. At eighteen years of age, with a 32E-24-35 figure, I appeared on 330 mammoth posters with the slogan, 'It's time to let my bra make an impact'.

'Kelly fitted the bill perfectly,' said the sales and marketing director, Malcolm Vagg, at the time. 'She's the right age, attractive, naturally big-busted and she knows what she wants from a bra.'

Interestingly, that was one of the only ranges available to voluptuous women at the time, and though it was notably prettier than anything else on the market for girls my size, it certainly wasn't the kind of thing I'd choose now.

right: Launching my lingerie range for New Look in Paris in October 2006.

In just a decade, British women have caught up with the French when it comes to stylish under-garments. My first Triumph campaign was before the days of Agent Provocateur and the lingerie revolution, when most women bought their undies in M&S, a job they saw as a chore rather than a treat. If we managed to wear a matching set of bra and knickers it was deemed good going, and if it wasn't grey and tired-looking, that was even more impressive. If you were bigger than a D-cup, you really didn't have much choice and had to wear what you were given, and more often than not that was something even your granny wouldn't be seen dead in.

Think how much times have changed – now women of all sizes have the most incredible choice of lingerie: even good old M&S has smartened up its act and sells a range of styles and colours designed to make women feel sexy, alluring, feminine, sporty, or however you want to feel.

Six months after that first campaign for Triumph, I signed a new contract to appear on the world's largest bra billboard. Triumph were really pleased with the public reaction to the first campaign, and wanted to continue using me as the face of their Flaunt collection. Measuring about 30 metres in height and 18 metres wide, the billboard was put up above the M4 flyover as you headed into London from Heathrow, and again attracted loads of media coverage, especially as between the two campaigns I'd done my somewhat controversial stint on *The Big Breakfast*, which meant I was better known to the public. There were even complaints from motorists, who said that other drivers were slowing down to take a longer look at the massive poster and causing traffic jams.

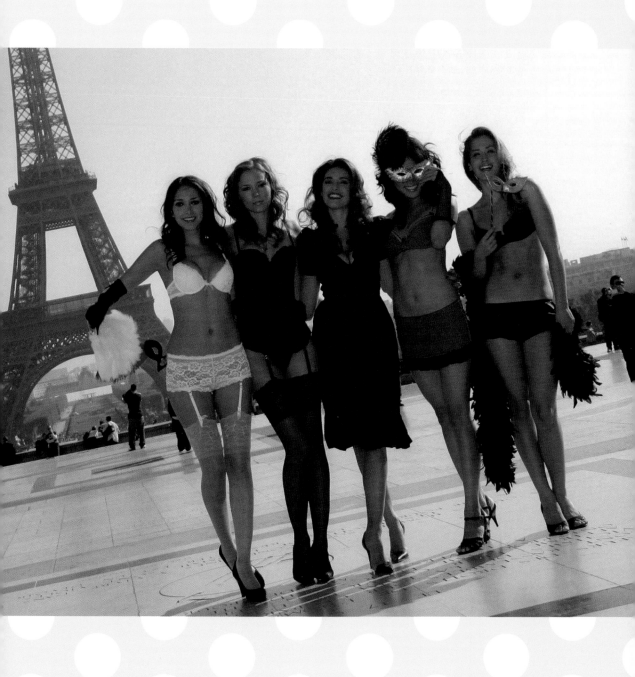

night-time style

15

What I love about being a woman is the variety of options available for us to wear when we go to bed. For example, we can choose from slinky silk-satin nightgowns, flirty tulle baby doll negligées, classic cotton men's-style pyjamas, Victorian-inspired broderie anglaise nightdresses, or simply Marilyn Monroe's favourite: a squirt of Chanel No 5.

Every girl has days where she wants to go for the comfy, cosy option – the crisp, cotton androgynous pyjama – and I love them. I have them in plain white and simple striped shirting, and they're what I enjoy wearing when I'm lounging around at home before bedtime. Contrary to popular opinion, men also seem to love girls in classic PJs – they're not threatening and I think they like the contrast of something that's traditionally designed for men against the curves of a woman's body. It's a bit like the 'woman in a man's suit' thing, and it seems to drive men wild.

You don't have to spend a lot of money to get decent pyjamas, many of the high-street chain stores and mail order companies do good ones, but I do recommend going for 100 per cent cotton. Natural fibres are definitely the best option for sleepwear, as they're the most comfortable in terms of maintaining body temperature and allowing your skin to breathe. The summer version of the classic PJ – wearing cotton boxer shorts with a simple ribbed singlet – is also a brilliant option. Once again it has that unisex appeal that can look very alluring on a female body.

opposite: Sometimes all you need to create the right effect is a simple white shirt.

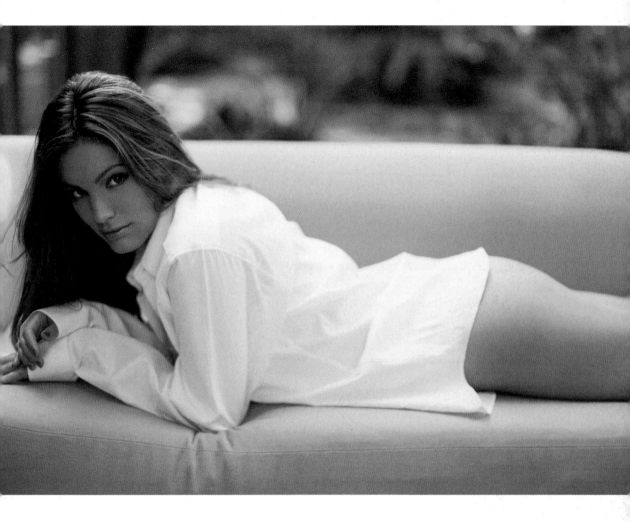

What is important at bedtime – and I don't necessarily mean 'in the bedroom' when I say 'at bedtime', since dressing for the bedroom can be a whole different ballgame – is that you don't wear anything restrictive. Comfort is imperative, but that doesn't mean you should be a slob, so no tight tops or underwiring – never wear a bra in bed – and no synthetic fibres, unless they're the new, breathable ones like microfibre, which is kind to the skin.

If you get cold in bed, natural fibres are best: silk is renowned for its thermal qualities, so if you can get silk jersey pyjamas, you're on to a winner. If you do tend to get chilly at night, I recommend wearing cotton flannel or silk jersey nightwear, then using blankets on the bed to create more layers of trapped air, which equals insulation. It's never good to turn the heating up and sleep in a room that's too warm: it's much healthier to have a cool room temperature and snuggle into cosy bedclothes.

right: Don't rush to turn off the lights; subtle lighting can be incredibly flattering.

Despite my penchant for classic pyjamas, there's definitely a place for more glamorous nightwear, especially if you're going away on a romantic break with a lover. Again, luxurious natural fibres are key if you're going to be intimate: light-as-a-feather silk chiffons, smooth-as-butter silk satins, delicate handmade lace and silk ribbons are all far more sensual than scratchy old polyester and nylon.

When the time comes for seduction, don't rush to turn off the lights. OK, so you don't want a fluorescent strip light illuminating the bedroom, but subtle candlelight can be incredibly flattering. If you're ready to get intimate, you should revel in the fact that he wants to be with you and enjoy the confidence this should bring with it. Remember, men rarely notice the bits women are self-conscious about – he's interested in the sparkle in your eyes, the smile you break into when he pays you a compliment and the way your body responds to his, not the couple of extra pounds you think you gained in the last fortnight or the tiny bit of cellulite on your thighs.

Feminine charm is at its best when you maintain an air of mystery, so take some time to master the art of undressing. Whether you undress for your man or he undresses you, take it slowly and enjoy discovering what lies beneath, and remember to wear beautiful, soft-to-the-touch clothing that feels good against the skin, such as velvet, cashmere, angora or satin.

Unless your lover suffers from an inferiority complex – i.e., he's smaller than you when you're wearing your favourite shoes – leave your heels on till the last minute. I've yet to meet the man who doesn't love seeing a near-naked woman in heels, and they have the added bonus of making your legs look longer and slimmer, as well as making you stand taller, metaphorically speaking, which always gives a bit of a confidence boost.

Don't go overboard with perfume though: even a light spritz can be a turn-off to men, who tend to prefer women *au naturel*. However, I do think there is something incredibly seductive about freshly bathed, delicately scented skin. So, if you have the chance, enjoy a long soak and use a lightly fragranced moisturiser or body oil before getting dressed.

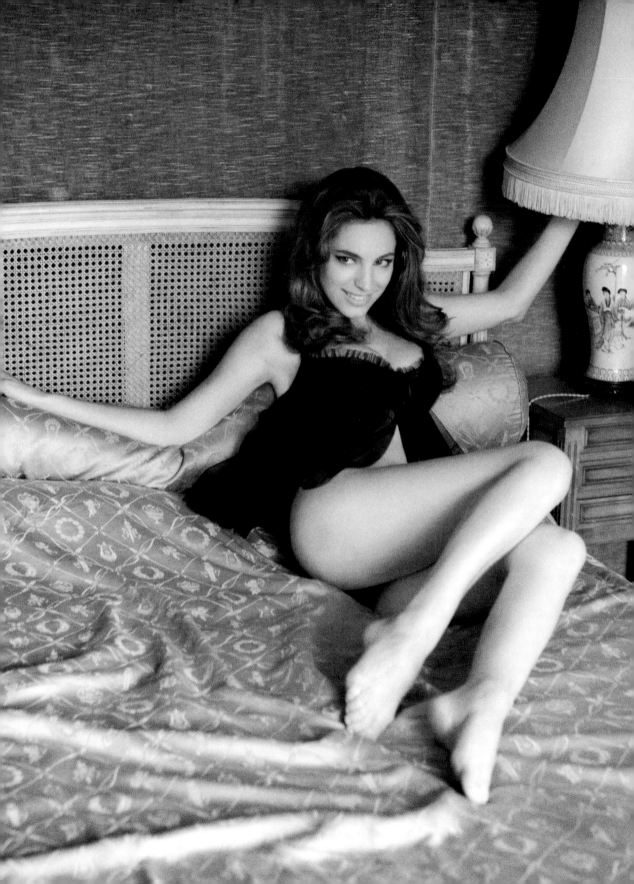

' a girl in like havin pistol on table – the wrong w but it's ha thinking

bikini is
a loaded
our coffee
e's nothing
th them,
rd to stop
about it "

Garrison Keillor

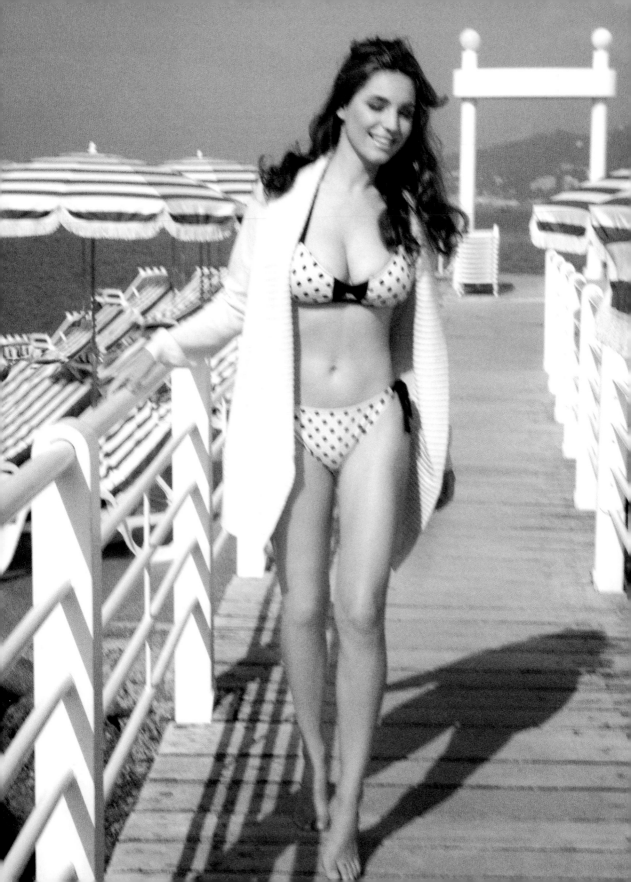

the bikini:
what's all the fuss about?

16

Most women have worn a bikini at some stage in their lives, and I have probably worn more than most. This most simple of garments – and let's face it, it is only a few triangles of fabric strategically strung together – has played a leading role in my career, and in many happy memories throughout my adult life.

I did my first bikini shoot when I was sixteen years old, perching on the side of a friend's boat in Kent. I was wearing a red string bikini with white piping, which I bought for about £20 in a shop called Laura Jane in the West End. I vividly remember the day I bought it. It took me a while to find a style that fitted well, because my bust is much larger than my bottom, so I'd usually have to resort to buying two different-size bikinis and discarding one half of each.

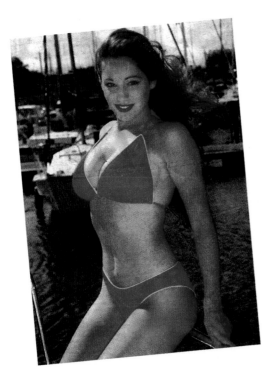

When I found this one, I was thrilled and bought it in loads of different colours – brown, green, red and blue – because it was so flattering. I ended up wearing them on loads of photo shoots, and they travelled around the world on holiday with me for years.

I've worn bikinis for modelling assignments, in films, for TV presenting and on holiday – in fact, I love bikinis so much I've even designed my own collection. But I was merely following in other people's footsteps, as two-pieces have been worn for hundreds of years. In fact, there are wall paintings as far back as 1400 BC, of Romans and Greeks wearing bikini-like two-pieces for athletics.

left: The first bikini shoot I ever did, aged sixteen, on a friend's boat.

Despite this early evidence of bikini-wearing, it wasn't until the latter half of the twentieth century that the bikini was considered civilised attire for 'nice ladies'. In the 1920s, Parisian burlesque dancers and showgirls used to wear a version of the bikini, but it still wasn't considered genteel, and in America it was portrayed as positively shocking. In fact, if you think about it, it's pretty much an excuse to wear a bra and knickers in public.

In 1930, the Americans introduced something called the Hays Code, which regulated strict dress codes and behaviour for actors and actresses on the silver screen, and said the navel couldn't be exposed in films. Can you imagine how limiting that would be? I think it's fascinating how our sense of what's acceptable has changed in such a relatively short time – just think, when many of our grandparents first watched movies there was still strict censorship.

Fairly typically, it was the French who refined the two-piece and put it on the fashion map. Two Frenchmen are credited with 'inventing' what we know and love as the bikini: Jacques Heim made what he called 'the world's smallest bathing suit', which was known as the 'atome', or 'atom'. Heim was inspired by the two-piece costumes worn by American former beauty queen and actress Dorothy Lamour, Jayne Mansfield and other Hollywood starlets of the era, including a young Marilyn Monroe.

But it's a French motor engineer called Louis Réard, whose father owned a lingerie shop, who is credited with giving the bikini its name. He used about 75cm of fabric to make an even tinier garment than Heim's, inspired by the women he had seen sunbathing in St Tropez. His design proved just as explosive as the atomic bomb testing that was taking place at Bikini Atoll in the South Pacific at the time, so he decided to give his design the same name. Réard unveiled his newsprint bikini to an unsuspecting world in July 1946 by flying planes trailing the message, 'Bikini, smaller than the smallest bathing suit in the world.'

Little did he know what a commotion he was about to cause! The revealing nature of his design caused outrage in certain circles, and he couldn't even find a model to wear his creation in a Paris fashion show, because everyone was afraid of the scandal that would surround the wearing of 'le bikini' in public.

"the atom bomb of fashion"

A strip-dancer called Micheline Bernardini, who worked at the Casino de Paris, eventually agreed to model his newsprint halter-neck design, with high-heeled peep-toe cork wedges – it's a look I really love and you can see where I get some of my ideas from.

The famous fashion editor Diana Vreeland apparently described the bikini as 'the atom bomb of fashion', and another Paris fashion writer said it was like seeing a woman emerging tattered from the blast. It's not quite how I think of this lovely ensemble, but there you go...

In America, women were escorted from beaches if they were caught wearing a bikini, the Belgians wouldn't allow them and the Pope banned them in Catholic countries. They were even too much for the supposedly liberal, laid-back Australians. For many years – right up until the 1960s, in many places – wearing a bikini was frowned upon by the moral majority: it simply wasn't considered suitable attire for a respectable girl.

How times have changed: today you could wear less to a nightclub and still be allowed in. It took a long time for the world to accept the bikini, though – over a decade, in fact – which I think is a great shame, as it's a really fun, flirty piece of fashion. I can't imagine not being able to wear a bikini on the beach or for a photo shoot. It would be such a waste of a great garment.

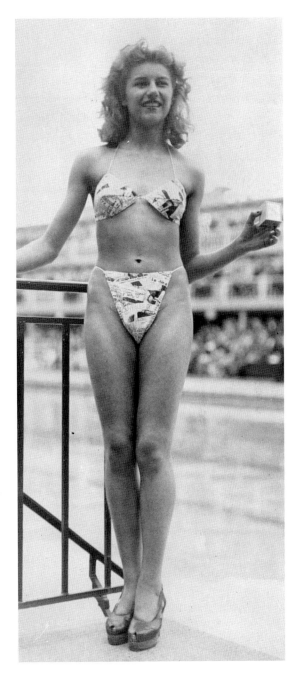

right: Michele Bernardini models Louis Réard's explosive newsprint bikini in 1946.

In the early 1940s, the bandeau-style
bikini top started to become fashionable among
forward-thinking – or should I say rebellious? –
young women, inspired largely by a photo shoot
in *Life* magazine. It featured a model called Chili
Williams, who became known as the 'Polka Dot Girl'
after appearing in a white strapless bandeau bikini
top and what I can only describe as matching
hotpants-style shorts with big red polka dots.

She looks gorgeous in that all-American
pin-up style I love, with her golden blonde curled hair
and bright red lips curved into a beaming smile. This
pose was an important development in the accep-
tance of the bikini, though it's rumoured that the
magazine received over 100,000 letters from readers
in response to the picture – I'm not sure whether
they were letters of outrage or appreciation, but
I know which mine would be.

One woman who championed the
bikini and made it fashionable in Europe was
Brigitte Bardot, who used to parade her curves on
the beaches of the Cote d'Azur in the kind of bikinis
Louis Réard would be proud of. Although she initially
shocked fashionable society with her risqué
ensembles, it wasn't long before other young
women followed suit and the south of France
was awash with gorgeous young girls in bikinis.

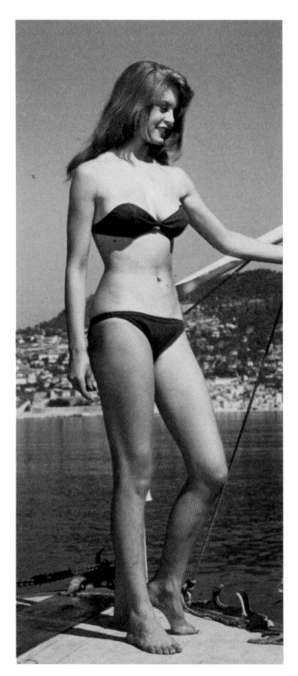

right: Eighteen-year-old
Brigitte Bardot raises the
temperature in 1952.

As early as 1952, an eighteen-year-old BB was being photographed for publicity shots in a narrow, boned bandeau top and skimpy briefs. What was the name of the film she was promoting? *Manina, La Fille Sans Voiles*, which was later renamed *The Bikini Girl*. Even then, in the early days of her career, before she became a platinum-blonde starlet – she had already been modelling for a number of years and apparently appeared on her first magazine cover at the age of fourteen – she looked impossibly glamorous.

Another fabulous Bardot bikini moment was in *And God Created Woman*, a 1955 film shot by her then husband, the director Roger Vadim. Cavorting on the beach in a gingham two-piece, she was the blonde bombshell of every man's dreams. Who wouldn't want to be that?

I love Brigitte Bardot's playful sex-kitten image. She has a girlish charm that's sexy without being predatory or intimidating and she's really inspired me to enjoy wearing bikinis as she always looked so natural and comfortable in them. For years after making *The Bikini Girl*, Bardot revelled in the title, adopting it as her own and continuing to appear in the garment that had made her famous.

Towards the end of the 1950s, she adapted her bikini girl look to suit changing fashions, swapping her bandeau tops for underwired halternecks, which gave more cleavage and uplift.

In 1964, by then a fully fledged blonde star, she appeared on the cover of *Paris Revue* magazine in her trademark sultry bikini pose that made men want her, and women want to be her. With tousled hair, smoky eyes and pale, pouting lips, she is photographed, sunglasses in hand, almost as if she's been caught unawares, turning towards the camera. She looks absolutely gorgeous, in a carefree, sensual kind of way, and it's a style that's very hard to emulate, though a girl can but try. Although my colouring is completely different to Bardot's, I have tried to capture the essence of her allure in some of my photo shoots: that childlike innocence, combined with a knowing sexuality.

The same year, Bardot was photographed – I think to celebrate her thirtieth birthday – wearing an underwired bikini with a beautiful straw picture hat to cover her sea-dampened locks. Even with minimal make-up, she looks utterly fabulous, and is a constant source of inspiration for me.

Throughout the 1950s, America, which, as is still the case today, has a more conservative take on life than Europe, was still uncomfortable with the idea of wearing a bikini in public, despite its growing popularity across the Atlantic. However, Americans did welcome the appearance of an array of pin-up girls, who were photographed initially in fairly modest bikinis, featuring structured bra styles and generous, sometimes skirted bottoms, that gradually became more daring as time passed.

this page: Esther Williams inspired the photo shoot for my New Look bikini range.

opposite: By the early 1960s Sandra Dee was still displaying a wholesome image in her bikini. But all that was soon to change.

Esther Williams, the pin-up who swam her way to celluloid stardom, was a popular poster girl of the time, who had very outspoken, old-fashioned views on what was appropriate attire for a woman. 'Young girls can wear a couple of Dixie cups and a fishing line if they want, but that's not my lady,' said Williams. 'A bathing suit is the least amount of clothing you should wear in public, so you'd better give it some thought. A bikini is a thoughtless act.'

I must admit to admiring Esther Williams's style: she was the Ginger Rogers of the swimming pool, making synchronised swimming glamorous and earning herself the nickname of 'Million Dollar Mermaid', after the title of one of her films. Although she didn't succumb to the allure of the bikini, I love the fact that she made bathing suits so glamorous, with her beautifully styled hair and pin-up role. I often turn to her films for ideas, as we did for the launch of my swimwear collection. Although the styles aren't the same, you can see how we were influenced by what she did.

In contrast to Esther Williams' demure style, Bunny Yeager – winner of the 1947 'Florida Trailorcoach Queen' beauty pageant – was determined to promote the bikini, launching her career as a swimwear designer and photographer alongside her modelling work. Although frowned upon by middle America, she was hugely influential in powering the bikini into the spotlight of the masses. She would make flirty two-pieces in all shapes and styles from scraps of cotton, trimming them with flowers, rope, ribbons or whatever took her fancy, then she'd either shoot self-portraits or photograph gorgeous young models wearing her creations. These were the kind of accessibly girl-next-door pin-ups that popularised the bikinis among the masses across America.

Then, in 1960, Brian Hyland's 'Itsy Bitsy Teenie Weenie Yellow Polka Dot Bikini' was a chart hit, turning the bikini into a piece of pop culture iconography. I love the fact that someone wrote a song about the bikini, and how some poor girl was too embarrassed to wear it out in the open. The lyrics say so much about how people felt about wearing a bikini in public. At first, the girl in the song won't come out of the locker room, and when she eventually does, she covers herself up with a blanket, and then when she goes into the sea she begins to freeze as she daren't come out again as she'd have to walk along the beach in her bikini.

Some of that old-fashioned innocence can still be seen in some of the photographs of that period. For example, Sandra Dee was one of the most popular personalities of the time, yet it was still quite controversial for a wholesome American star to be photographed in such a revealing number.

It's amazing how little things had changed since the time of Chili Williams twenty years earlier. Sandra Dee might have been able to reveal a lot more flesh, but essentially there's the same pin-up styling, a similar Doris Day hairdo and a flirty look in her eyes, without looking like she'd do anything she shouldn't.

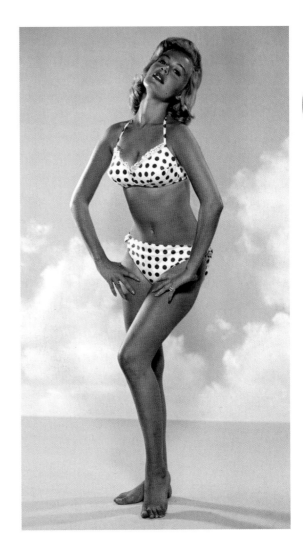

Likewise, Annette Funicello wore a very
modest bikini, with pants Bridget Jones would have
been proud of, in *Bikini Beach*, one of a series of films
that kicked off the beach movie genre in Hollywood.
Treading a fine line between implied sexuality and
wholesome acceptability, teenagers across America
started to find role models their parents were
comfortable with.

As the Sixties progressed, bikinis became
all the rage, signalling a more liberated lifestyle
across the Western world. It was the time of sex,
drugs and rock'n' roll: women were enjoying a new
sexual freedom after the arrival of the birth control
pill and the bikini was just another way to express
this carefree approach to life. The midriff was *the*
erogenous zone of the Sixties, with women rolling
down their bikini bottoms to show off their bare
stomachs.

Ursula Andress caused millions of men's
hearts to flutter when she emerged from the surf
as Honey Ryder in the 1962 Bond film, *Dr No*. It just
goes to show that sometimes a more substantial
style can be just as sexy as a skimpy little number. As
I've learned over the years, allure comes in what you
don't show, rather than baring all, and it's all about
confidence. Andress's bikini wasn't actually a very
flattering cut and it didn't fit her that well, either,
but she carried it off with such panache and
sensuality that all you remember is how great
she looked.

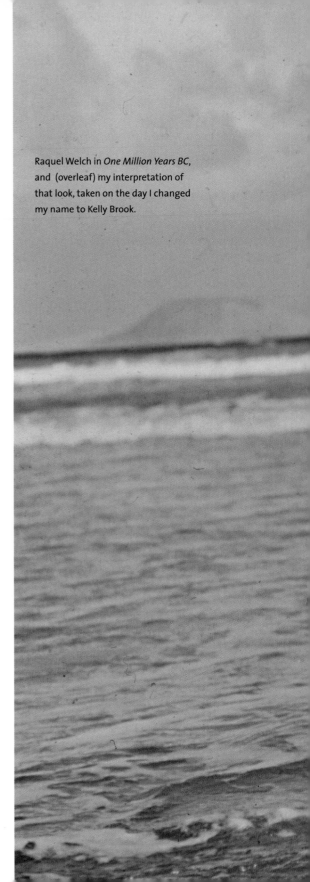

Raquel Welch in *One Million Years BC*,
and (overleaf) my interpretation of
that look, taken on the day I changed
my name to Kelly Brook.

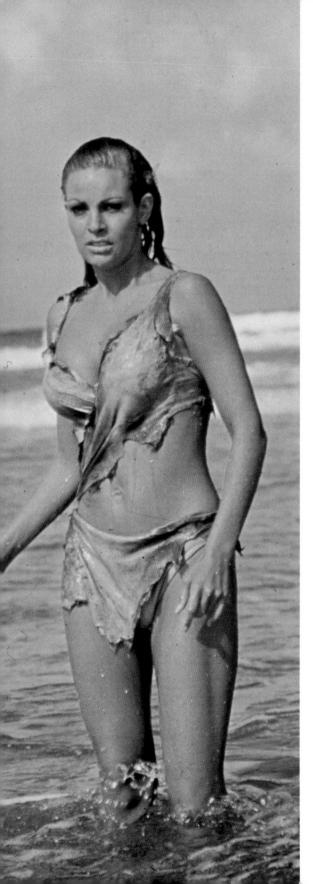

One of my favourite bikini babes was the Mexican-American actress Raquel Welch, who made a habit of appearing in swimwear throughout her career, first in one-piece costumes and later, as the bikini became more acceptable, in two-pieces that changed shape according to her film roles and fashion. The only constant was that she looked a million dollars in every single one of them.

One of her most famous outfits was a bikini of sorts: that fabulous cave-girl chamois leather bra and loincloth, with matching boots, in the 1966 film *One Million Years B.C.* I guess it's partly iconic because it shows what an early bikini might have looked like and although it's quite modest in terms of the amount of flesh it shows, it's still unbelievably sexy.

Hers is an image that's always inspired me, and was the inspiration for my first shoot with the legendary glamour photographer Jeany Savage in 1998 when I was only eighteen. Gary Cockerill, a make-up artist friend of mine who I've worked with for years, introduced me to Jeany, who had just discovered and launched the modelling careers of Melinda Messenger and Katie Price (Jordan).

We met briefly at a photo studio in Camden, north London, and right from the word go I really liked her, as she's very down-to-earth and bubbly. Her reaction when we met was 'F**k me. You've got big tits. You'll have to do topless.' She sent me off to the hairdresser's, where they cut my hair and gave me blonde highlights, all in preparation for my first shoot with the *Daily Star*.

On the day of the shoot, Gary gave me a Raquel Welch-inspired hairdo and make-up, and the stylist, Marcella Martinelli, sat in the studio cutting up strips of chamois leather to replicate that famous cave-girl bikini. Someone once asked Raquel Welch about the costume she wore, and she said, 'Between takes I took out some scissors, snipped away at the costume, and just kept on snipping. It also shrunk because of being continually soaked in the sea. There wasn't much to begin with and I really had to watch it to keep it on at all.'

Believe me, I know how she felt!

At the end of the shoot, Jeany rang the newspaper, who were creating a story to go with the pictures, and while she was on the phone, she barked across the studio, 'Kelly, what's your full name?' When I said, 'Kelly Ann Parsons,' she looked horrified and told the person on the phone that she'd call them back. For the next few minutes we discussed various possibilities and half an hour later, she rang them up and gave them my new name – Kelly Brook – and that's how I got my professional name.

Not surprisingly, my friends and family were quite shocked when I first appeared in a national newspaper as Kelly Brook, wearing nothing but a skimpy home-made bikini that barely covered my modesty, but once the photos were published, my phone didn't stop ringing with bookings for modelling assignments: I'd never worked so much.

The other photographs of Raquel I love are the ones of her wearing a brown halterneck bikini with a ring detail, which were taken in the late Sixties for *Vogue*. For me, the images perfectly capture the way that newly liberated women were able to flaunt their sexuality with confidence. She embraced her femininity and revelled in it: where Brigitte Bardot was coquettish, Raquel Welch was raunchy.

For me, Raquel is the ultimate bikini babe, with her curvy 37:22:35 silhouette, topped off with that fabulous full mane of chestnut hair and the smouldering make-up. I often ask my hair and make-up team to do a Raquel Welch look, and this is what I mean when I say it. It's proper, full-on womanly glamour, but still natural enough to feel real and gorgeous – it's not that plastic glamour you see so much these days, and I think a lot of men would agree with me.

In the 1970s, women on Copacabana Beach in Rio de Janeiro, Brazil, started to wear tanga-style bikini briefs – or thongs as they're often called – which revealed their neat little bronzed buttocks to the world, setting a trend that was to spread to beaches everywhere, with varying degrees of success, depending on the shape of the wearer's bottom!

In 1974, the American fashion designer Rudi Gernreich, who encouraged topless sunbathing when he created the monokini a decade earlier, launched his version of the thong, with Giorgio di Sant'Angelo airing his version – though how it could have differed much, I don't know – a year later. Both were featured in trendsetting magazines such as *Vogue* and *Sports Illustrated*, which is unbelievably influential when it comes to swimwear trends, especially in America, but, understandably I think, the public was cautious about adopting the look *en masse*. In the Eighties and early Nineties, thongs and G-strings were popular in some areas, but I can see why they aren't for everyone.

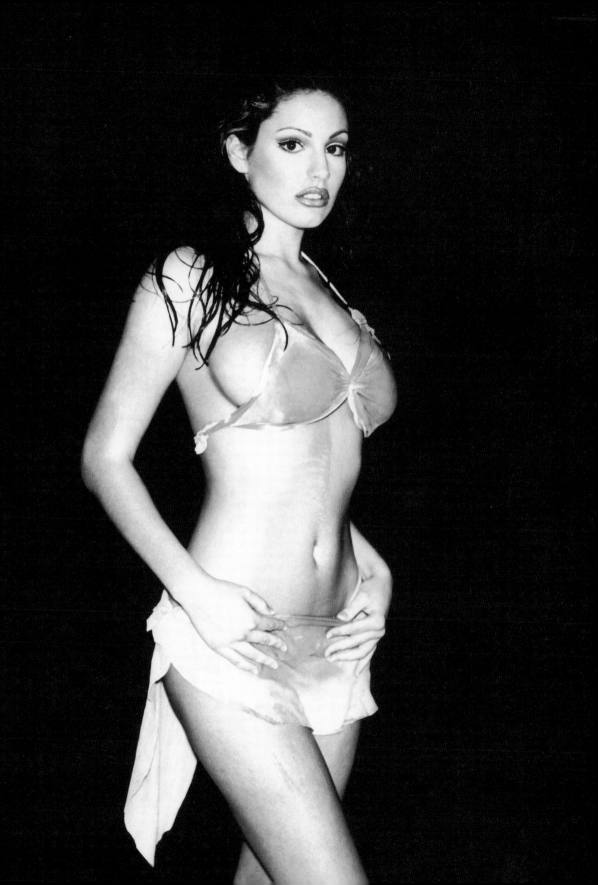

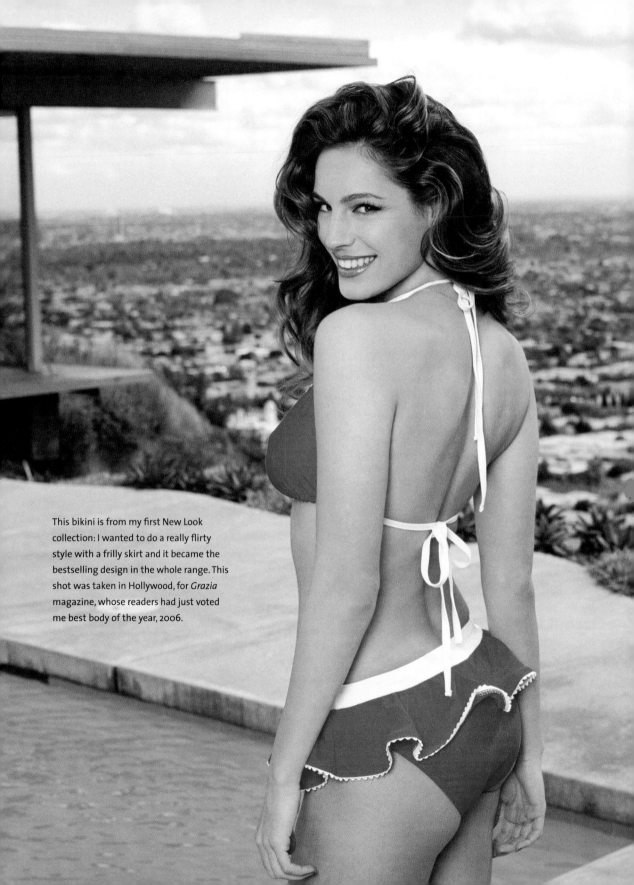

This bikini is from my first New Look collection: I wanted to do a really flirty style with a frilly skirt and it became the bestselling design in the whole range. This shot was taken in Hollywood, for *Grazia* magazine, whose readers had just voted me best body of the year, 2006.

how to look your best in a bikini

17

When it comes to choosing a bikini to suit you, take a look at icons with a similar body shape to yours – hourglass, pencil, pear-shaped, athletic, etc. – to find styles that suit you. If you're curvy, look at the bikinis worn by the likes of Raquel Welch and Brigitte Bardot, or for more contemporary styles, Claudia Schiffer and Pamela Anderson. For those with a more athletic shape, check out the looks worn by Elle Macpherson, Cindy Crawford, and for boyish styles turn to Jemima Khan or Kate Moss for inspiration.

always buy a flattering size

If possible, look at ranges where you can buy the tops and bottoms separately, as women are rarely the same dress size above and below. Don't worry about size and what it says on the label, just go for the one that looks good and feels comfortable, so it will give you confidence.

My tip is to try tops that are one size smaller than you would normally buy as they'll give you a good shape and impressive cleavage – but don't squash yourself into something much too small or you'll just end up looking awkward.

fit style to shape

If you're busty, avoid excess frills and flounces, which can make you look even bigger than you already are. The exception to this is frilly knickers, which can look flirty and cute even on a voluptuous derriere. I think skirted briefs look fabulous, too, and have a glamorous retro pin-up feel to them. Sometimes, you just don't want everything hanging out, and they feel incredibly feminine – when I designed my first swimwear collection, the skirted styles were the bestsellers in the range.

Try on a selection of different styles – you might be surprised by what suits you. Some styles look shapeless on a hanger, but turn out to be immensely flattering once they're on.

I was once told that if you have big boobs you should avoid draw-string bikinis and wear underwired styles instead, but I've found that the classic triangular drawstring style can be incredibly flattering, whereas fitted, full-cup styles often make me look even more enormous. If you're large and going for a structured top, try a balconette style that's uplifting and support-ive without looking like you've trapped two balloons in a sack. Halternecks are usually flattering if you have a larger bust, but strapless is rarely a good look. It's just as important to wear supportive fabrics as it is to go for the right cut. Look out for Lycra®, which adds stretch.

If you're petite up top, strapless, bandeau styles are often flattering, as are athletic-style sports bikinis. While if you have a slim, boyish figure, go for complementary boy-cut pants or a classic brief.

right: I love the cherry print detail on this bikini, which I was wearing for a shoot in Malibu in 2001. It reminded me of the dress worn by Marilyn Monroe in *The Misfits*.

pick your palette and patterns

Use colours to highlight your assets – if you're proud of your cleavage and would rather draw attention away from your lower half, wear darker bottoms and a lighter top.

Use pattern in the same way – it goes without saying that horizon-tal stripes create an illusion of width, and vertical stripes add length or height – use this trick if you're pear-shaped – it's great for balancing out smaller boobs if you wear a horizontally striped top with vertically striped bottoms.

Have fun with pattern: I think bikinis are one of the few ways you can be a bit cutesy as a grown woman and get away with it. I love colourful, childlike prints like cherry or banana designs – very Carmen Miranda.

Likewise, use design details to draw the eye to the parts of your body you're comfortable with and away from those you're not. So, if you're the owner of rather generous buttocks, it's probably best not to wear a bikini with a slogan or design on the back of the bottoms. But if you have a fabulous décolletage, draw the eye to it by wearing a top that fastens at the front with a jewelled or beaded clasp.

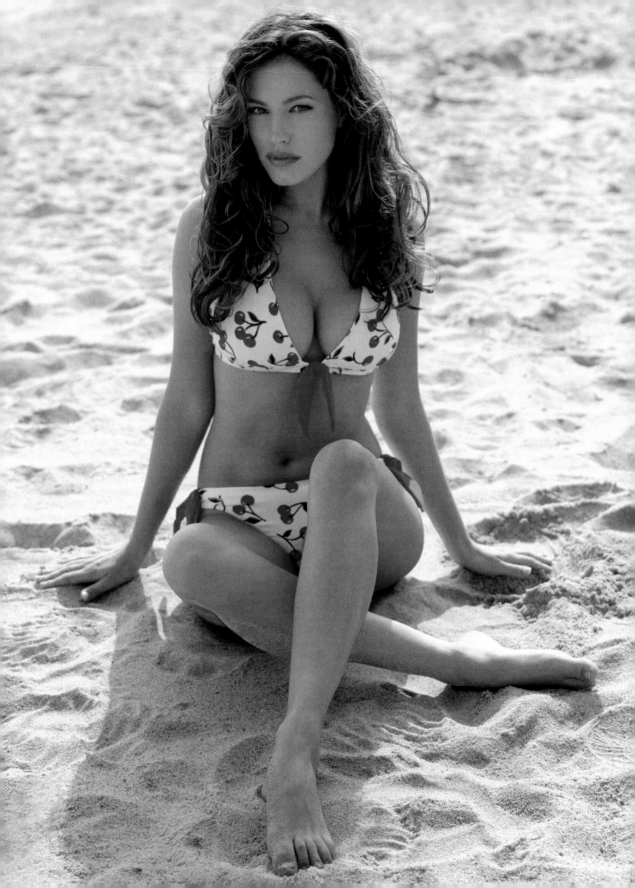

Wear colours to flatter your skin tone. I prefer classic, bold colours on pale skin, such as navy, red or apple green, and black, white, browns and khaki can look lovely on olive or bronzed complexions. It's definitely worth taking a few bikinis away on holiday, so you can adapt your wardrobe according to the depth of your tan.

choose a bikini that suits your needs

I know it might sound silly, but when you're choosing a bikini, consider what you'll be doing when you wear it. If you're really sporty and love waterskiing, diving and water parks, then a flimsy little, sequinned number should be left on the rail, or at least kept for a day when you're exhausted and just want to flop. Likewise, if your goal is to get a great all-over tan, don't choose the high-fashion bikini with criss-cross straps and asymmetric cut-outs everywhere.

Thongs are perfect for sunbathing and getting an almost all-over tan, but no matter how great your body, they're never the most flattering style, especially when you're walking around. I suggest that if you want to wear a thong for sunbathing, carry a matching sarong, so you can pop that on if you're going for a walk.

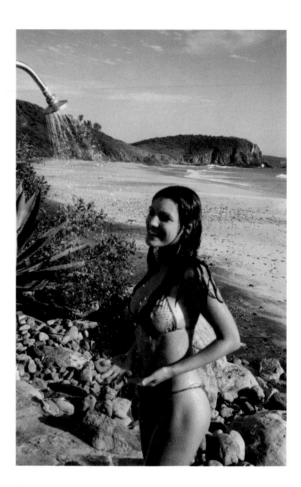

and finally...

Remember, one bikini is never enough. There's nothing worse than putting on a damp bikini if it hasn't dried out overnight, or having to make do when you've spilled ketchup at lunch. These days, you can buy fantastic bikinis on the high street or the internet, without having to spend a fortune, so even the most frugal holidaymaker can afford a capsule bikini wardrobe.

Once you've chosen the best bikinis, then the next task is to make sure that you look at your very best when you come to put it on. And for this there is one key rule: preparation is all. So here are a few ways to ensure your body looks bikini beautiful when you hit the beach.

Pilates is a great way to tone your body, lengthening your muscles and flattening your midriff. I also recommend hiking in the hills, swimming and riding your bike, all of which I love doing. For me, exercise has to be about having fun in the fresh air, rather than being a grind you really hate, and what I love best is just dancing.

Avoid alcohol and caffeine for a fortnight – or a month if you can bear it! – before you go on holiday. It can cause water retention and bloating, which isn't going to make you feel your best when you slip into a bikini on the first day of your holiday.

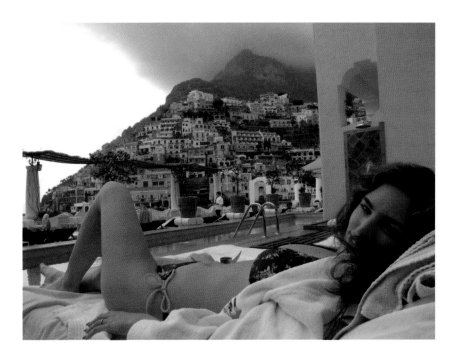

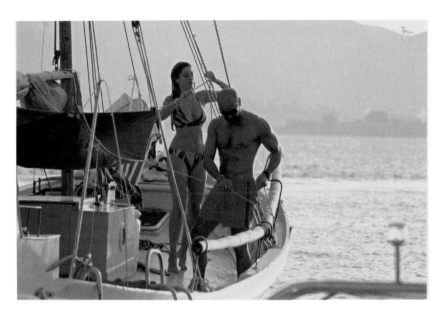

left: I love this shot of Billy and me on holiday in 2005, aboard a Greek fishing boat in the Mediterranean – I'm wearing a Missoni halterneck bikini.

Exfoliate and moisturise regularly in the lead-up to your trip, so your skin is in tip-top condition and prepared for sun exposure. Remember to use a good high-factor sun cream to protect your skin, though. Burnt skin is never a good look! I'm a big fan of body scrubs and I regularly go to a Korean spa, where they scrub me all over, then apply fresh ginger to the skin. You feel a bit sore for a while, but the results are amazing.

I think **pale skin** is very attractive, but if you want some colour when you first venture out in your holiday bikini, book in for an all-over spray tan a couple of days before you depart.

Remember to **wax** a couple of days ahead of a tanning treatment, and at least a couple of days before you plan to wear a bikini, so that any irritations have time to settle down. Personally, I like to be completely fuzz-free on the beach.

I always have a **manicure and pedicure** the day before I head off on holiday: ugly hands and feet can ruin a beach body.

Sometimes I have **lash extensions** before a holiday: the salon applies individual fake lashes alongside my own, which makes them look thicker and saves me wearing mascara while I'm away.

Don't have your hair coloured or chemically treated in any way immediately prior to a holiday in the sun as prolonged exposure to the sun and chlorine can wreak havoc with your hair, leaving it looking exactly how you didn't want it to. Try to have any colour done at least a fortnight before you go away, so it has a chance to settle first, or wait until you return home, so your hairdresser can use the right products to condition and ensure your locks are in tip-top condition.

Stay hydrated – both on the beach and on the flight out to your destination. As well as drinking plenty of water on the flight, avoid alcohol. I use a moisturising masque the day before flying and a water spritzer with a little lavender rose during the flight to stop my skin drying out.

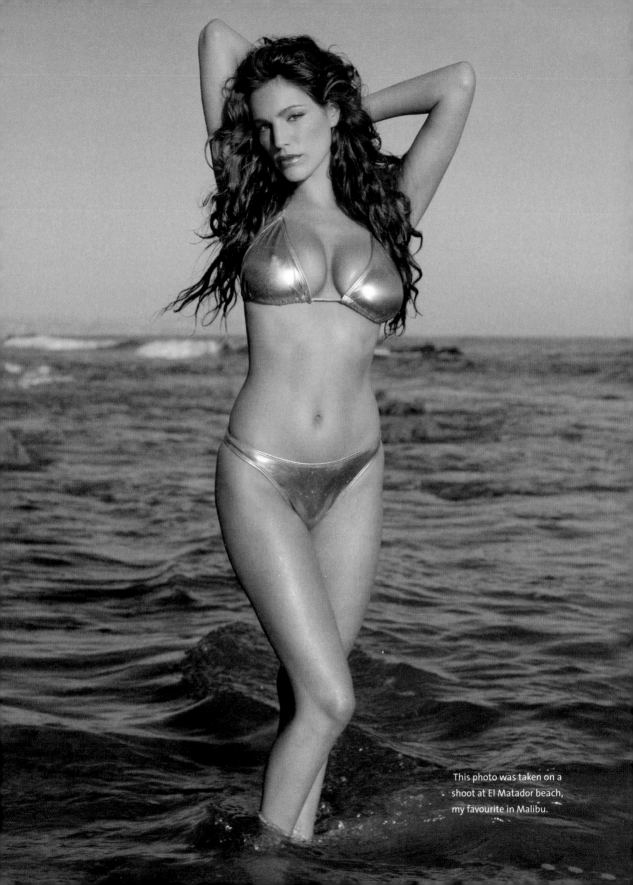

This photo was taken on a shoot at El Matador beach, my favourite in Malibu.

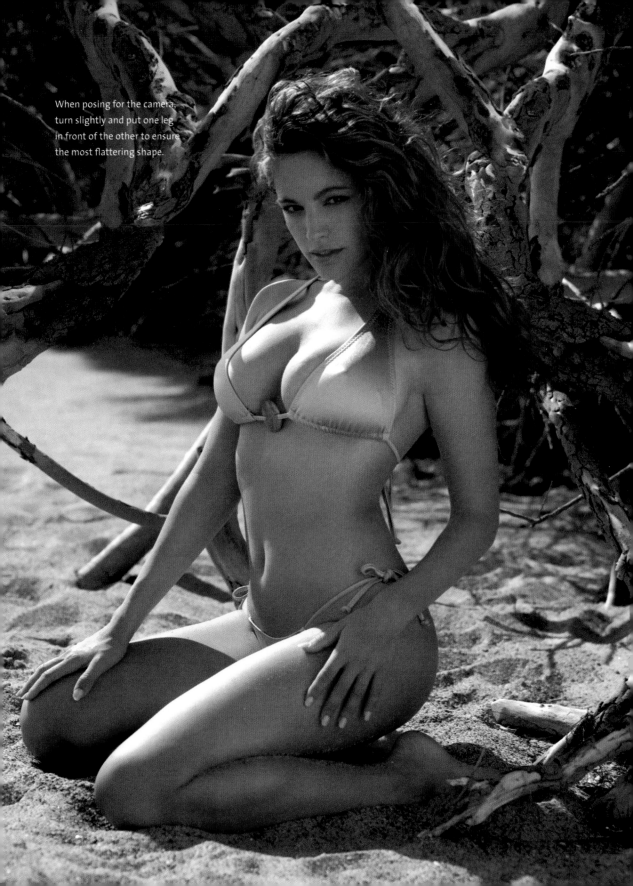

When posing for the camera,
turn slightly and put one leg
in front of the other to ensure
the most flattering shape.

strike a pose: tricks of the trade

I've had a lot of experience modelling swimwear over the years, and spending so much time being photographed in the nearly altogether has taught me a thing or two about how to strike a pose and look my best in minimal clothing. Here are my tricks of the trade for looking great in a bikini on camera – secrets every woman should know.

1 It's always good to turn slightly when posing for a picture, so you're not front on, offering your widest silhouette to the camera. Even the slimmest women tend to twist on a diagonal when they're facing the camera, while turning their face into the lens. That way, with your shoulders back and your stomach held in, you get to show off your bust and butt rather than your front-on silhouette, which is rarely the most flattering shape.

2 Always wear high heels to give you posture, even if your feet aren't in shot. Wearing heels throws your body into a more feminine stance than flats, as well as giving the illusion of longer legs.

3 The classic pin-up pose is to put one leg in front of the other, slightly bent, as it elongates and narrows your silhouette.

4 I hate armpits in pictures so tend to avoid having my arms raised if I'm having my photograph taken. It's easy to get caught waving or reclining on the beach, so just be careful.

5 Don't sit or kneel upright front on, so you have two stumpy knees facing the camera. Always turn, so your legs are slightly side on to the lens, which is far more flattering.

6 No one is symmetrical, so figure out which is your best side and offer it to the camera.

7 Keep your chin down slightly, but don't allow shadows to creep onto your face.

8 Backlight is always flattering, so ensure the light source is behind you rather than blasting your face. Flashlight is rarely flattering, but standing by a window can throw a lovely soft light on your skin. Early morning and early evening are what is known in the photography world as the 'magic hours', when the sun is low and glowing, and we always do outdoor shoots at dawn or dusk. Try to avoid having your picture taken in the harsh midday sun.

9 Use eyedrops to make your eyes glisten.

10 Visiora body make-up is great if you're being photographed in a bikini or swimsuit as it covers blemishes and stretch marks, and Screenface – a professional make-up artists' store in London – is the only place in the UK you can find it.

11 This is a tip I learned from synchronised swimmers: paint gelatine in your hair while you're swimming, then when you wash it out afterwards, your hair will be really soft.

12 I've got really small stubby nails with a very short nailbed, and if I'm doing a shoot, I'll have acrylic nails added to make the nail bed look longer as it looks much nicer in photos. I go to Zoe at Daniel Galvin's London salon.

13 I always have a pedicure before a photoshoot. Try not to use too much colour, though: buffed feet with shiny, healthy-looking toenails look so much prettier than hard skin and unloved nails, which often lets British women down.

14 If you've got a nice smile, flaunt it when you're having your photo taken: there is nothing better or more attractive. Always think about something that makes you happy and it will come across in the picture – think of the man you love, or a place you enjoy spending time, that way there'll be a little intrigue in your eyes and you won't just be staring at the camera with a false smile on your face. If you feel like you've been posing for ages and your grin has become fixed, change your expression. Above all, be natural – no one smiles all the time – or think of something that amuses you.

Unless you're seriously comfortable with your look, avoid being photographed on the beach at the beginning of your holiday when you won't have a tan and can't rely on make-up to cover up the fact. Wait until the end of the holiday, wash your hair, put on your favourite bikini (or a costume, sarong or kaftan if it makes you feel more comfortable), pop on some waterproof mascara, and if you feel you need it, a light sunscreen foundation or bronzer to even out your skin tone. After that all you need do is smile.

15

part two: my style

195

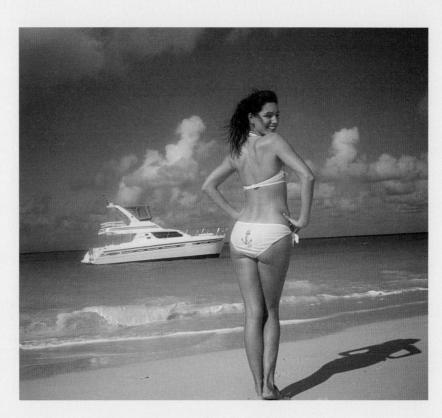

Here I am in Agent Provocateur on holiday in the Turks & Caicos in January 2007. My friend Lisa and I chartered a yacht for a few days after I finished the Lynx shoot in Miami. I think the anchor design on the bum is great – really cute and cheeky! No wonder there's a smile on my face.

The final key ingredient to looking great in a bikini isn't actually to do with what you wear, and how you get into shape, but is all about what you take with you onto the beach. As so often, it's all about being prepared so that you can relax and enjoy yourself. These are the things I would always recommend that you take with you:

● I love to buy a cheap classic straw basket when I arrive at wherever I am staying: it gets me into the holiday mood instantly, and I use it as my beach bag for the rest of my stay but am not upset to part with it when I leave as usually, by the end of my holiday, it looks like it's seen better days.

● If I haven't brought a hat with me – and I don't usually bother, as they're awkward to pack – I'll try to buy a lovely straw sunhat to shade me from the sun. Not only do they look really pretty, they cover up salty beach hair a treat.

● I never wear jewellery on the beach, except a small pair of stud earrings or some huge gypsy-style hoops, which I think look really stylish with a bikini. Rings, bracelets and necklaces just leave marks – likewise, watches – and who wants to monitor the time when you're on holiday, anyway?

● A good pair of sunglasses is crucial when it comes to looking stylish on the beach: not just to protect your eyes from glare, but to give you that important touch of Hollywood glamour. Try on lots of different styles before you buy to find one that suits your face shape and don't just go for the fashionable shape of the moment – a timeless classic that suits you is a much better investment.

● A couple of sarongs are a really useful addition to any holiday wardrobe and I always carry one in my beach bag. They're perfect to wear as a cover-up when you go to the pool bar for lunch, as a dress, or even as a headscarf if your hair is looking less than perfect. Depending on the fabric, you can roll one up and use it as a head support on your sun lounger, or even use it to dry yourself if you're caught short without a towel.

● I love kaftans on the beach: they're very Liz Taylor and super glamorous. If you're heading to Morocco or the south of France, you should go for bejewelled bikinis and fabulous flowing kaftans, while in Ibiza or the Caribbean, I'd suggest a simpler look.

● I like to have a couple of books with me for holiday reading, plus my iPod   I love chilling out on the beach to stuff like Café del Mar.

● I carry a tube of conditioner in my beach bag and put it in my hair before I go in the sea as it makes your hair easier to detangle and stops helps prevent it getting too damaged. I always try to have a fresh-water shower as soon as I can after going in the sea, too, to avoid the drying effects of salt water on my skin and hair.

● I always have some Elizabeth Arden Eight Hour Cream in my beach bag: it's a great all-round skin balm for soothing dry patches, makes a good after-sun if your skin has been a little overheated, soothes chapped lips and helps maintain supersoft skin on dry areas such as elbows and knees.

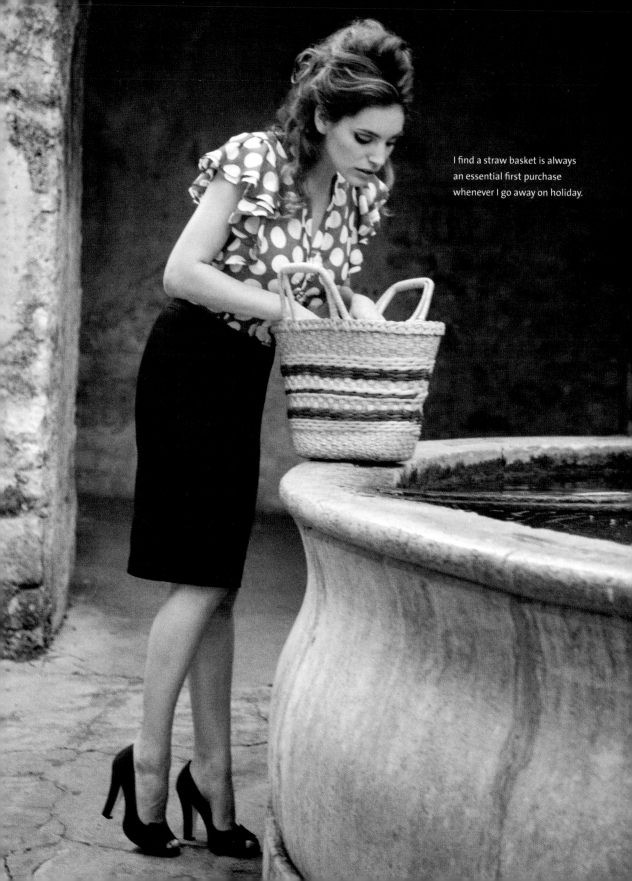

I find a straw basket is always an essential first purchase whenever I go away on holiday.

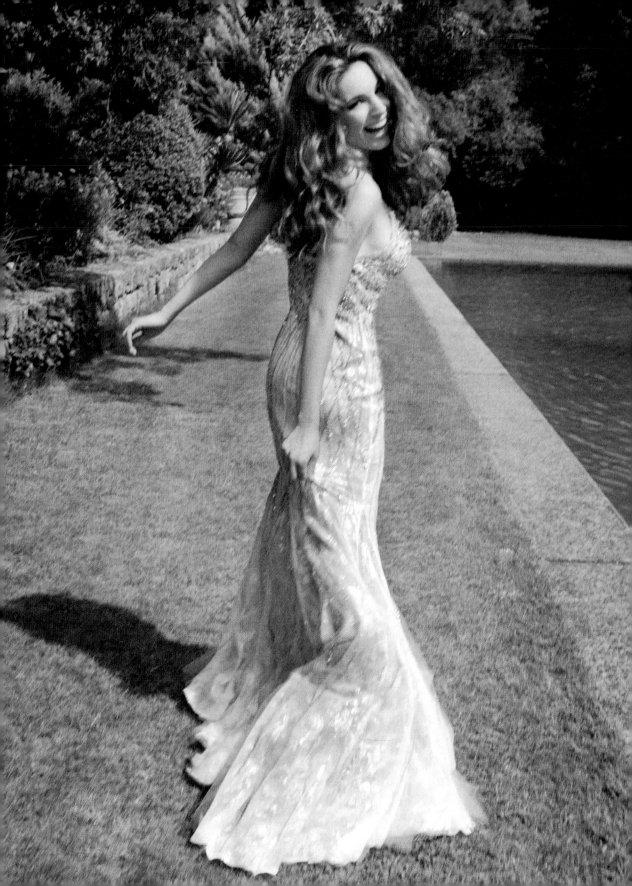

dressing up and weekend style

For me, dressing for a big occasion is about looking the best you possibly can. It's about making an effort and making the most of your assets in a timeless, elegant way. I tend to book myself into the hairdresser for either a blow-dry or sophisticated up-do that's reminiscent of old-time Hollywood. I believe that if your hair looks fabulous, you'll walk taller and have a smile on your face, and it's definitely a key ingredient to looking great for a big night out, whether you're attending the Oscars or the office Christmas party!

I also like to make sure my make-up is just so. I enjoy wearing make-up and am comfortable with very dramatic looks, but not everyone is, and if you don't *feel* right, you'll be fidgety all evening, so make sure you're at ease with whatever look you are wearing.

It's also important to balance hair, make-up and your dress. They have to work together, not fight each other, so try to create a complementary, cohesive look that works overall. Sometimes, all you'll need is a coat of mascara and a slick of lip gloss, while at other times your outfit might call for full-on smoky eyes and red lipstick. If you're unsure, ask someone you trust for their opinion, and give yourself time to adapt the look if you still aren't convinced.

When it comes to party dressing, I adore wearing vintage gowns and beautiful, well-made evening dresses by designers who really know how to cut for curves, such as Bellville Sassoon, Vivienne Westwood, Roland Mouret and Marchesa. I need structure in my eveningwear – there's no way you'll find me in a slinky bias-cut slip dress – and an important part of choosing glamorous attire is establishing what works for you in terms of silhouette, colours and styling, then adapt your choices accordingly. That's not to say you shouldn't try different looks from time to time, but don't succumb to the latest fashions if they just don't suit your body shape/colouring/taste.

left: I love dressing up for the big occasion.

weekend style

Even the most glamorous women like to dress down when they're off duty. Although I adore wearing pretty dresses, high heels and fabulous make-up, there are days when we all like to slip into a pair of jeans, a cosy sweater and our favourite, comfortable boots, and I am just as susceptible to the charms of easy everyday clothes as the next person.

When Billy and I are hanging out at home in the Kent countryside, walking in the hills near our LA home or visiting his parents in Chicago, I'm happy to adopt a casual wardrobe that doesn't ooze feminine glamour. Quite honestly, I love lounging around in my slippers, or wellington boots if I'm outside, though I confess there are certain criteria that are still important to me. I love my clothes to *feel* fabulous, so shoes or boots have to be really comfortable or I may as well be wearing heels! I can't bear nasty synthetic fabrics next to my skin, so if I'm wearing a sweater, I like it to feel baby-soft – and yes, I do love cashmere.

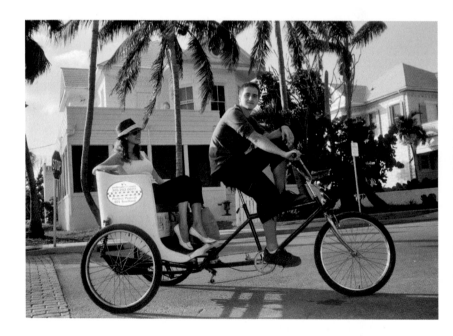

right: Travelling round Key West in a rickshaw.

opposite: Relaxing in Key Largo.

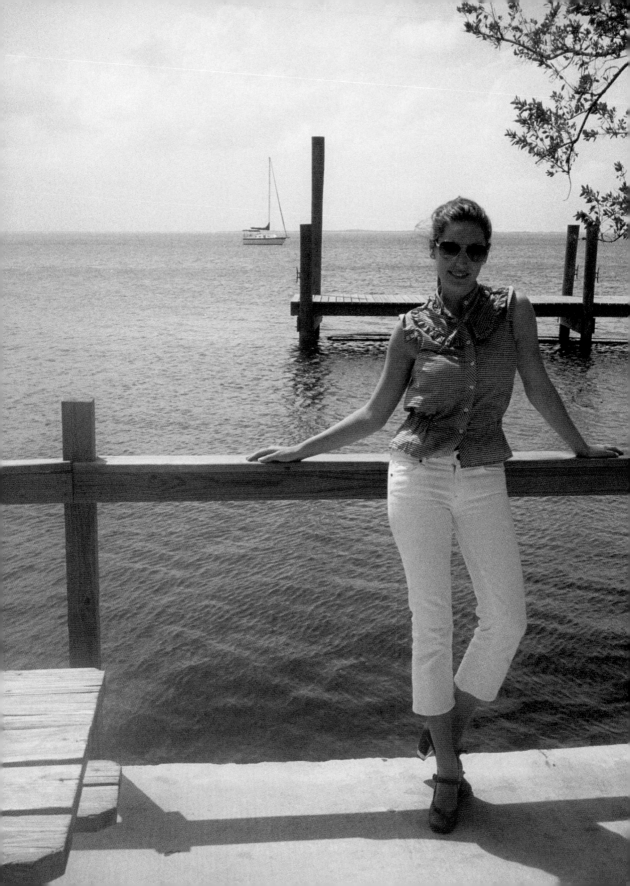

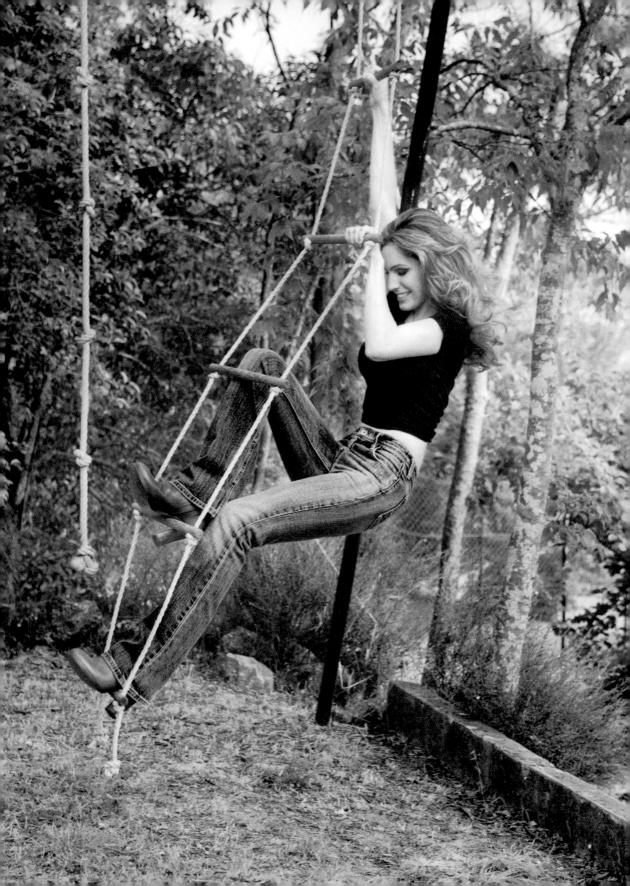

right: Enjoying the New England fall in Lennox, Massachusetts, while wearing my green A-line belted coat by Dries van Noten and a flat tweed cap borrowed from Billy.

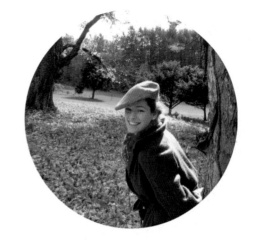

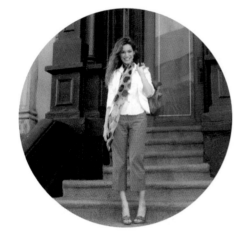

above: At an audition in Hollywood: the addition of a printed silk chiffon scarf made a simple outfit a stylish one

Accessories are still important though. For example, even when I'm just wearing jeans and a roll-neck in the winter, I like to wear beautiful quality leather gloves and a stylish hat. I also have a soft spot for really stylish sunglasses – I'm not into wearing the latest fashionable style, I prefer a pair that suit my face shape and go with the rest of my outfit. I have a few pairs, mainly by Oliver Peoples, and I choose them according to the style of my outfit.

As I grow older and become more confident with my sense of style, I'd rather own a luxurious cashmere scarf or one pair of butter-soft lined leather gloves – my favourites are a pair of elbow-length green Céline gloves that cost me a fortune, but I know I'll wear them forever – than go into a high-street chain store and buy loads of tat that will fall apart within weeks. Accessories make the lady.

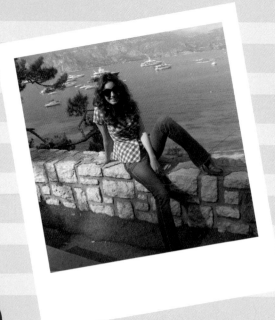

Taking a stroll around Cap d'Antibes, on the French Riviera, in a pair of Paper Denim & Cloth jeans and a Vivienne Westwood shirt and boots.

holidays and travel

I love the chance to play with clothes when I'm on holiday, adapting my wardrobe to my temporary surroundings. While I always remain true to myself and try to wear styles that suit my body and colouring, it can be fun to adopt some of the culture and fashion of your destination.

For example, when I'm in Italy, I adore wearing chic Capri pants and knotted shirts with ballet pumps, or feminine full skirts, all of which are reminiscent of the great Italian sex kittens of the 1950s, such as Sophia Loren and Gina Lollobrigida. Many Italian women look just as gorgeous as these goddesses of the silver screen: they seem genetically programmed to look fabulous! I love films like *La Dolce Vita*, *Roman Holiday* and *The Talented Mr Ripley*, which show Italian style at its best.

When I was working in Fiji on *Celebrity Love Island*, I had a lot of fun wearing tropical print dresses and pinning flowers in my hair for that classic *South Pacific* look.

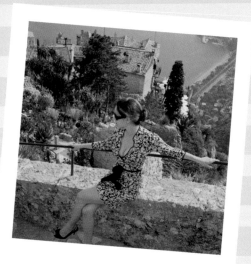

Wearing a printed Diane von Furstenberg wrap dress and peep toe, slingback heels while relaxing in Eze, France.

Wearing shorts and a midriff top at my favourite hotel in the world, the Villa Feltrinelli on Lake Garda, Italy.

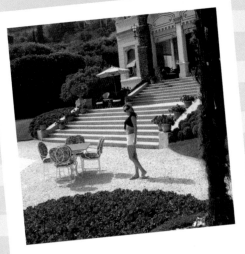

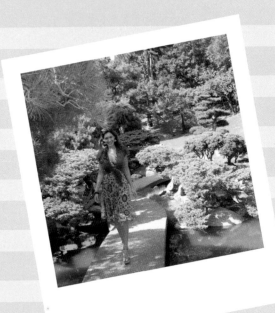

Walking around one of my favourite gardens, the Huntingdon Library in Pasadena.

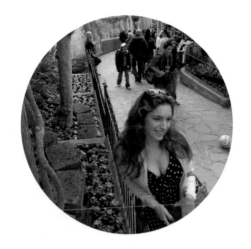

And when I've visited Morocco, I like to adopt the glamorous poolside style of Elizabeth Taylor: kaftans and jewels look fabulous – and you can always wear costume jewellery rather than real gems. In these ways, anyone can immediately feel more of a part of their surroundings – it can be really worthwhile.

Although many people think that relaxing on holiday means not bothering to put together a wardrobe, it is possible to look stylish without trying too hard. What could be less effort than putting on a dress? It's much easier to look good in a lovely dress than it is to put together a T-shirt and trackpants, because co-ordinating two pieces is more effort than wearing one.

"It can be fun to adopt some of the culture and fashion of your destination"

above: Shopping in Positano, Italy – one of my favourite holiday pastimes – in a Moschino polka-dot dress and a pink cashmere cardigan.

When I'm sightseeing or on the beach, I tend to wear pretty ballet pumps, Keds canvas plimsolls, wedge-heeled espadrilles or classic Brazilian Havaiana flip-flops, but I do love wearing heels when it's practical, though you try tip-tapping through cobbled streets in a pair of spike-heeled stilettos!

When it comes to make-up, if you can't be bothered, just pop on a little sunscreen, a slick of lip balm, and a pair of sunglasses – that's what they're for!

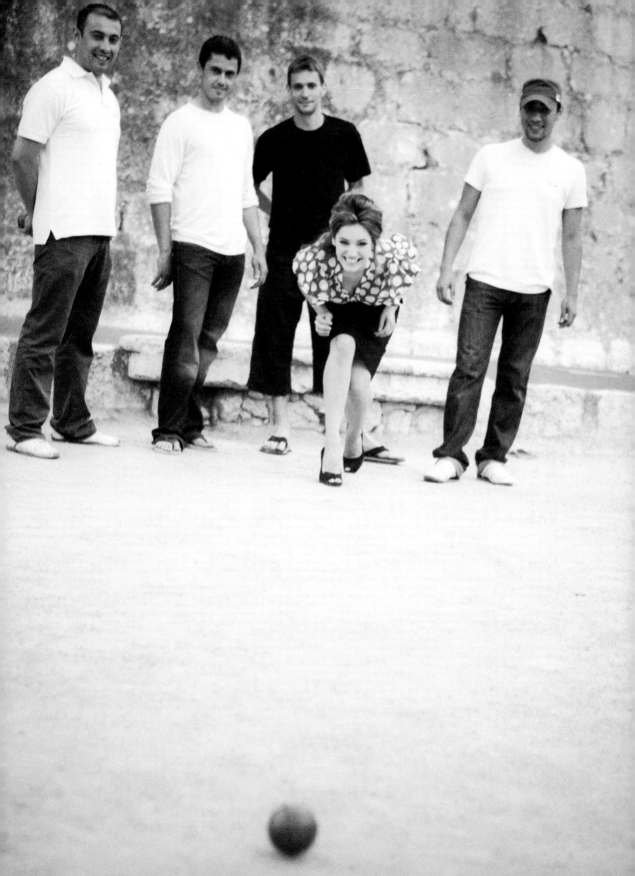

Kelly's capsule wardrobe

19

There are certain pieces in my wardrobe I consider long-term staples, clothes I can rely on to provide me with a classic style that suits me wherever I am in the world and whatever I'm doing. Of course they're not all I own – just like any woman, I add to them all the time – but they are the items I would feel lost without.

● Knee-high, black leather, high-heeled boots – mine are by Christian Louboutin

● A classic black bag. Mine's a Hermès Kelly bag. It's an expensive investment piece, I know, but it will never date and looks good with anything

● A black, belted knee-length trench coat – mine is made from grosgrain and is by American designer Derek Lam

● Sunglasses. I own several pairs, mostly by Oliver Peoples, in slightly different shapes, so I can choose the ones that best go with my outfit

● White tank-shaped ribbed vests, also known as 'wife-beaters'

● Pure cotton white shirts and mens'-style cotton shirting in simple stripes: I have styles by Paul Smith, Vivienne Westwood, Gap and Thomas Pink in my wardrobe

● Polka-dot blouses are a pin-up girl's essential. They're always feminine and fun and can be teamed with pencil skirts or jeans to add a little playful frivolity to an outfit!

● Breton T-shirts – very Brigitte Bardot

● Fitted, boot-cut jeans. They are classic, and even when they're not the height of fashion, they are always flattering

● Good-quality, slightly fitted plain white T-shirts from Petit Bateau, Gap, C&C California

● Capri pants – these are really sexy in the summer with espadrilles, cork wedges or ballet pumps

● Cashmere jumpers and cardigans. I like traditional round-neck styles in classic colours like white, baby pink and bright red. Best budget buys are from M&S, Gap and J Crew, but if you can spend a bit more try Ballantyne, Pringle and Brora

● Jersey dresses. Issa and DVF dresses are seriously flattering on a woman's body and great for travelling because they don't crease and are very comfortable. You can dress them up or down according to the occasion, by changing your accessories, make-up and hair

● Classic pencil skirt: I have them made by a trusted dressmaker, as well as styles by Alexander McQueen, Vivienne Westwood and Roland Mouret

● Neat tweed suits – I wouldn't be without a few of these classic suits with a pencil skirt and fitted jacket, preferably by Alexander McQueen or Vivienne Westwood

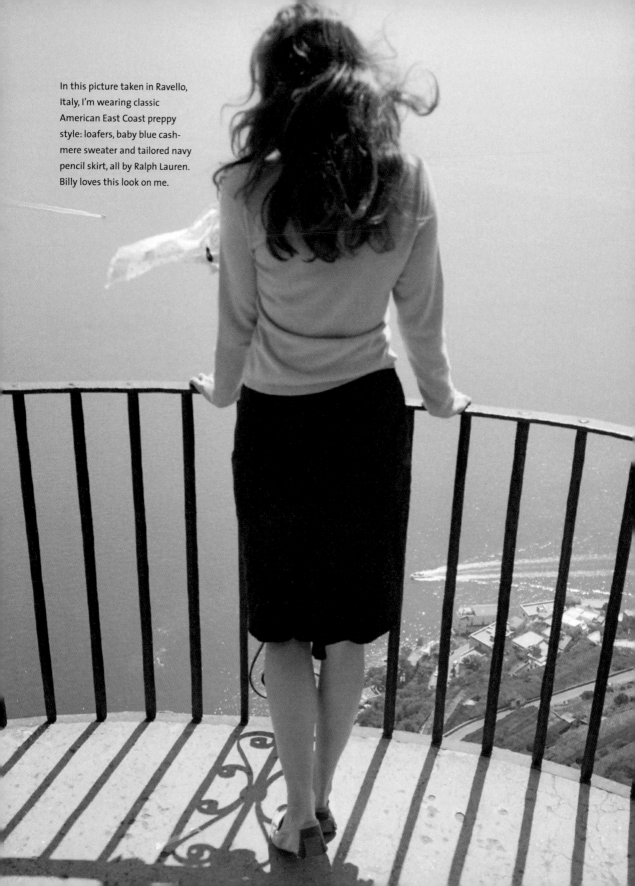

In this picture taken in Ravello, Italy, I'm wearing classic American East Coast preppy style: loafers, baby blue cashmere sweater and tailored navy pencil skirt, all by Ralph Lauren. Billy loves this look on me.

- Shift dresses: Moschino ones have a great fit and fun details such as bows or ribbons. They also do great summer dresses

- Short leather gloves. My favourites have a mink trim at the wrist and Holland and Holland do nice ones.

- Long leather gloves – I have a gorgeous elbow-length green pair by Céline

- Tights and stockings – black, matte opaque tights; flesh-tone fishnets and sheer black tights and stockings, usually by Wolford or Fogal

- High heels. One pair (at least!) each of black, red and metallic silver or gold strappy high-heeled evening shoes. My favourites are by Gina, Jimmy Choo and Christian Louboutin

- Havainas. While I'm a big fan of heels and the lengthening effect they have on your legs, there are times when only flats will do, whether you're going to the beach or just knocking around the house. For me, there's nothing more versatile than the classic Brazilian flip-flop, which I have in a rainbow of colours

- A warm, coloured winter coat. Mine is a lovely, A-line teal green coat by Dries Van Noten that can be worn loose or belted

- Long evening dresses. Mine are either vintage or by designers like Bellville Sassoon or Marchesa, who cut to flatter a curvy silhouette

- Short evening dresses. Again, I wear a lot of vintage pieces, especially prom dresses, but I also like styles by Marchesa, Alice Temperley, Zac Posen and Roland Mouret

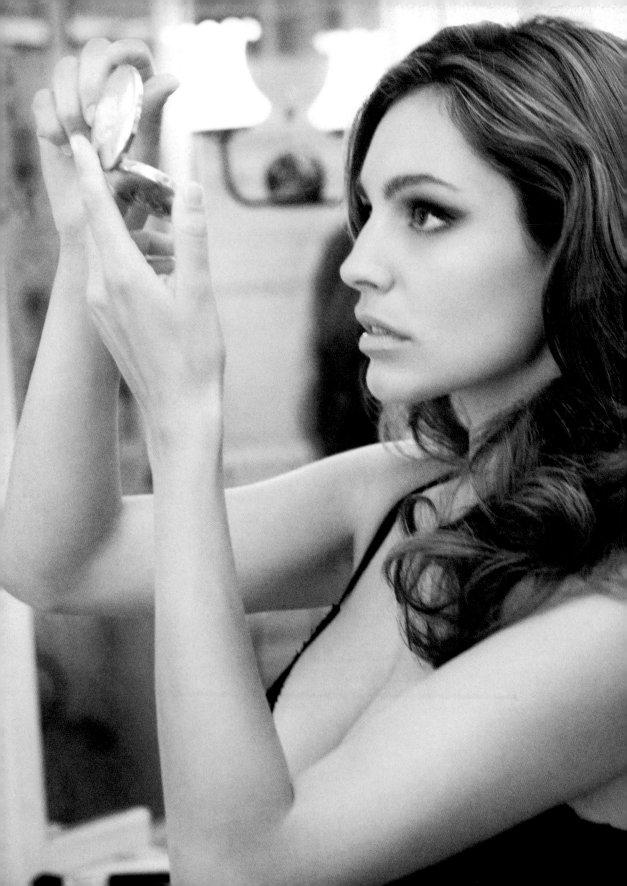

beauty queen

I absolutely love using make-up to create a certain look or add a little glamour. Whether it's a sweep of mascara and blusher or full-on 'maquillage', complete with red lips, false eyelashes, eyeliner and a dusting of powder, cosmetics are a powerful weapon in a woman's mission to be on the front line of femininity. From femme fatale to pouting pin-up, there's so much fun to be had with the contents of a cosmetics bag.

That's not to say you need to wear make-up every day; quite the contrary, in fact. I think it's lovely to see ladies looking fresh-faced and pretty in their day-to-day lives. During daylight hours, I think less is more when it comes to applying colour to your face – there's nothing worse than caked-on foundation and overdone eyeshadow in the harsh light of day. A dash of concealer, a lick of neutral lipstick and some brown mascara is often all that's required of a woman's daily make-up routine.

Some women are blessed with clear, even complexions and defined features that are naturally beautiful, without the need to enhance or refine with colour and shading. And most of us, if we take care of our skin and perform a little regular maintenance and groom-ing, can leave the house looking pretty good without applying more than a slick of lip gloss and mascara in the morning.

However, I do believe that many of us, armed with a few basic skills and a good kit containing the right products – and by that I mean the right products for you, not whatever's fashionable, expensive or new – can enhance and refine our natural beauty with the addition of some cleverly applied make-up.

It may be as simple as learning how to apply blush so as to create contours where they don't exist, or perhaps it's finding the perfect foundation to even out your skin tone. You might need to practise the art of applying liquid eyeliner to create that elegant cat's eye look that Sophia Loren made her own. However, with patience, most of us can master the small tricks of the trade that professional make-up artists use to flatter, alter and highlight your assets.

In ten years of modelling and acting, I have been privileged to work with some of the world's top make-up artists, who have passed on some of their knowledge and helped me understand my face. Although I frequently discuss using a certain style as inspiration – 'Let's do a Raquel look today', for example – the most important thing to remember is that make-up should be applied to suit *your* face. It's no good copying everything a friend does if she has completely different colouring and her face shape is round when yours is heart-shaped.

So, firstly I recommend getting to know your face. I know that might sound like common sense, but you'd be amazed at how many women have no idea about the structure of their own features or understanding of their skin tone and type. Once you have really started to understand what canvas you're working on, only then can you fully appreciate how to make the most of it.

If possible, spend some time with a professional make-up artist. Pop into your local department store, where you can usually book a session with one at some of the main brand beauty counters, the cost of which is usually redeemable against a purchase. Bobbi Brown, Laura Mercier and MAC are particularly good because they are brands devised by professional make-up artists and are very much about creating looks that work for individual women.

It's important to arrive without make-up on, and to be completely honest: tell them you want to learn how to make the best of your features and that you'd like some practical advice on application techniques. Don't be swayed into a demonstration of how to use their seasonal palette but suggest

that if you are to become a customer of their brand, you want to identify a capsule selection of products you can use and rely on regularly. When you're done, don't be pushed into spending a fortune on expensive products if you're not convinced. Suggest that you'd like to go and see the results in daylight and live with the look before you buy the products.

The long-term benefits of professional advice are incredible, and some well-known make-up artists even do private lessons. So the next time you splurge on a night out, a pair of shoes or a massage, think about how great you'd feel if you could apply your make-up properly and invest the money wisely. You could even suggest to your loved one that it might be something you'd like as a birthday treat.

Although there are no hard and fast rules when it comes to make-up application – much of it is about personalising techniques to suit you – there are a few tips and tricks I've learned over the years. They've been gleaned from those with far more experience than me, and will definitely help when you're refining your own techniques.

Many of my favourite looks are inspired by my movie star and pin-up icons. But just as when you draw on their wardrobe for your sartorial style, it's important not to blindly copy every detail; instead, make sure it works for you. Be quite sure a red lipstick is the right tone for your colouring, for example – so many women say they can't wear red lipstick when they just haven't found a flattering shade to work with their complexion.

right: Great make-up can change your look dramatically.

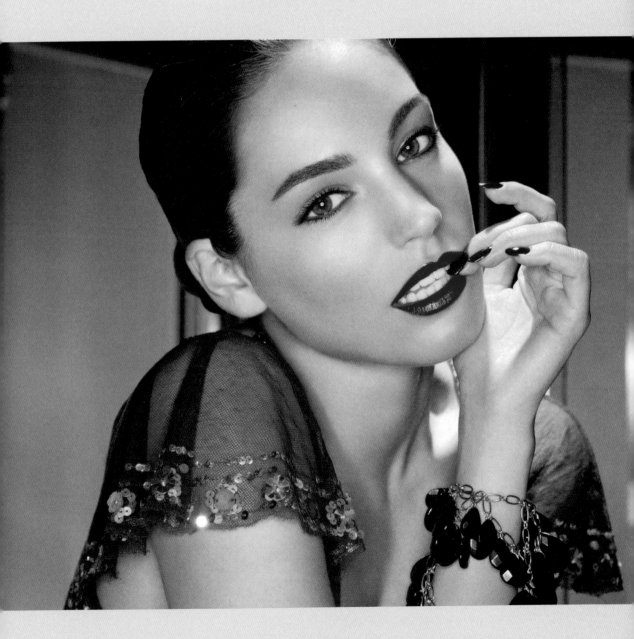

Kelly's make-up tips

Laying the foundations

Take your time finding a foundation that works for you: most companies produce samples, or will let you take home a tester to try in your own time. I was once told that foundation is one of the most expensive mistakes women make – because they try it under pressure in harsh department-store lighting and end up panic-buying the wrong shade. I'll bet you have a number of bad foundations lurking in your make-up bag or dressing-table drawer!

When you're selecting a foundation, it's really important to see it in daylight, and to ensure it blends with the skin on your jawline and neck, since this is the area it will have to meet without giveaway lines.

Unless you're wearing stage or television make-up, foundation shouldn't feel like a mask. You should be able to conceal blemishes and under-eye shadows using a good-quality concealer, then apply foundation as a light base for the rest of your make-up.

Rather than used an oil-based foundation, which can slide on the skin and settle in fine lines, most professional make-up artists suggest using a good moisturiser a short while before applying a non-oily foundation, even on dry skin. It's usually worth blotting with a single-ply tissue – just separate the layers of a standard tissue – once you've applied it to remove any excess oil, then use a light dusting of loose powder to finish.

Brow-beating

Eyebrows are so easily forgotten when women are assessing their face, yet they are possibly your most important feature because they help frame the eyes. They are also the easiest feature to change dramatically, which, if necessary – and some small modification is almost always beneficial – can make a huge difference to your appearance.

It's worth taking the trouble to groom your brows so they look tidy: when I was a teenager, my mum taught me to use tweezers to carefully pluck mine and it's really paid off. However, it's easy to overpluck and end up with straggly strips, so either have it done professionally, ask a trusted friend to do it, or at the very least take it slowly until you've got the hang of it.

Threading (using twisted cotton to pull out individual hairs) is another popular method of brow control used by many women, but it's best done professionally.

On a daily basis, it's worth using a brow brush to keep your brows tidy, and possibly a brow pencil if you need a little more definition.

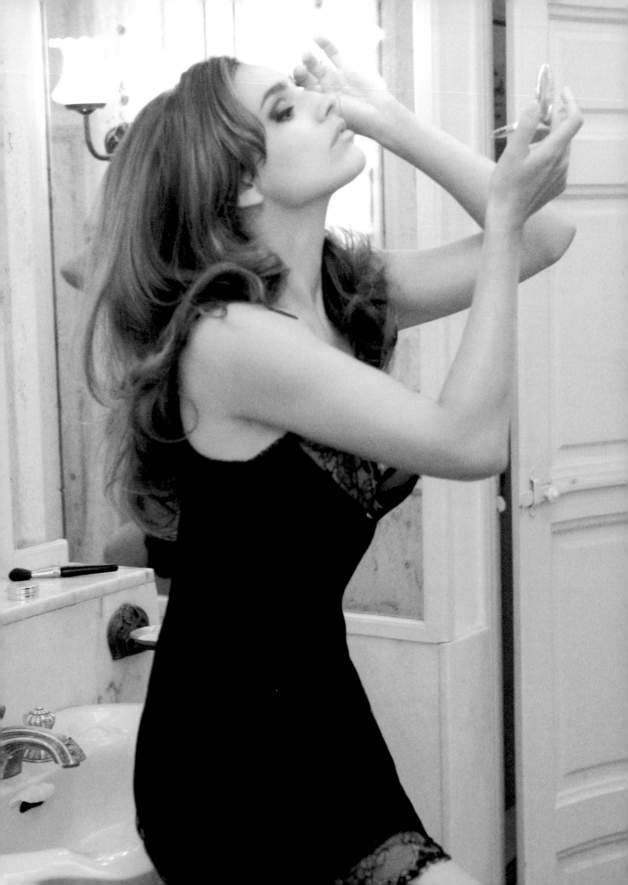

Eyelash tricks

One of my favourite make-up tools is my eyelash curler, which I was given when I first started modelling and have been recommending to girlfriends ever since. Though they look rather intimidating, they are actually very easy to use and can really make your eyes look 'wide open'. Always use them *before* applying mascara, though, as if you use them afterwards the lashes will be brittle and might break.

I think false eyelashes are one of the most undervalued cosmetic accessories available to women. Most women think they're only appropriate for showgirls and fancy dress, so they ignore their potential for subtly enhancing evening make-up. In our mothers' day, false lashes were not as sophisticated as they are now – nowadays you can buy individual lashes that can be applied to the outer edge of the eyelid, just to add some luscious length and depth. The trick is to add lashes gradually, using transparent lash glue – the black adhesive is a bit of a giveaway – and don't overdo it unless you want to go out looking like Liza Minelli in *Cabaret*!

Luscious lips

If your lips are dry, slick on a little Vaseline, then use a soft toothbrush to buff away dead skin. Don't be too harsh, though, you don't want to burn your lips, just give them a gentle exfoliation so lip colour glides on more smoothly and lasts longer.

Nailed on

Don't forget that your nails – fingers and toes – are all part of your personal presentation and should be styled to complement your overall look. The most versatile nail shape is neat, not too long and 'squoval' (square with rounded edges) in shape. And yes, I confess, I do use fake nails on occasion when I want some serious talons.

These are just basic guidelines to use as a starting point when you're trying to create looks inspired by classic Hollywood pin-ups. I often reference film stars or other style icons when I'm planning a look, sometimes working with a stylist and a make-up artist to achieve the results I want, other times doing my own make-up.

I think it's important not to be too literal when referencing styles from a bygone era: for example, if you're dressed in a 1940s-style suit with stack heels, be careful not to look like an extra from a period drama by going for too authentic a make-up look.

You don't want to look like you're wearing fancy dress, so personalise your ensemble by adding a contemporary twist, such as wearing sassy, modern shoes or wearing your long hair in a loose tousled style instead of a prim chignon. As long as you do something different to avoid a copycat, you should be able to carry off a retro style with panache.

When it comes to make-up, it's fun and stylish to use authentic techniques, just as long as you adapt them, and your colour palette, to suit your facial features. If you're going for classic make-up with a vintage outfit, just remember to show your originality another way, through your bag or shoes, say.

Here, I've outlined the basic techniques and colour palette used to recreate certain signature Hollywood looks I particularly like. I've also described how to achieve a hairstyle to complement each look, but you don't, of course, have to go for the whole shebang.

Get the look

Inspired by Marlene Dietrich and Greta Garbo, this is a very carefully defined face, with a pale, even complexion, narrow, arched brows and deep, dark blood-red cupid's bow lips. It's quite a tricky look to wear without seeming dated, but it can look particularly stunning if you're wearing a simple evening gown with sleek hair – the sultry German chanteuse Ute Lemper is the perfect example of someone who carries off this look in a contemporary way.

Make-up

● Use a concealer a shade or two lighter than your natural skin tone to eliminate any dark circles under the eyes and even out any blemishes or uneven skin tone. A pale, creamy complexion is the key to achieving this look. Apply a matte, creamy foundation, being careful to ensure a smooth, even finish, then use translucent loose powder with a large brush to complete your look.

● Eyebrows should be groomed so they are narrow and arched, then define them with a brow pencil if they're pale.

● For smouldering eyes, sweep pale ivory matte powder shadow across the whole eye socket, including the lid and brow bone. Use a matte steel-grey in the crease of the eye and black eyeliner on the lid, then use eyelash curlers and apply *two* coats of black mascara.

● Use a small sweep of pale, tawny-coloured matte powder blusher under the cheekbones to define the contours, being careful to avoid 'rosy' colour on the apple of the cheeks.

● Use a brick-red lipliner to create a neat, elongated cupid's bow shape and fill in with a deep blood-red lip colour. Blot with a single ply of tissue, apply a dusting of loose powder, then repeat the process for maximum staying power.

Hair

I think hair looks best worn sleek with this look, either smoothed back into a neat ballet dancer's bun or slicked into Marcel-style waves, which can be achieved using large rollers and setting lotion, then brushing the hair out smooth.

the *1930s*

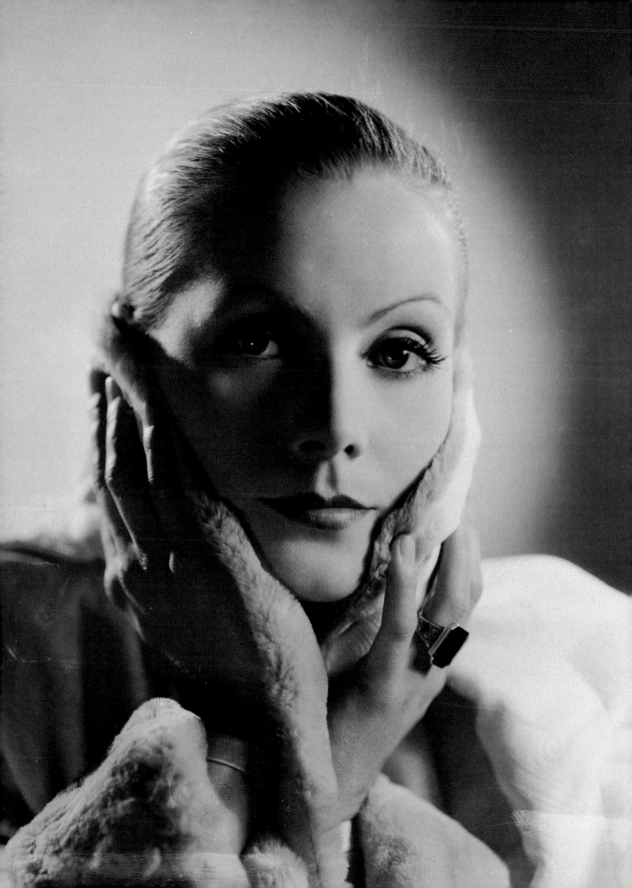

the *1940s*

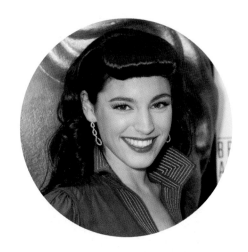

Get the look

I look to the irrepressible Bettie Page when I want 1940s inspiration, because she exuded a happiness and self-confidence that's rare today. She's a prime example of someone who was beautiful because of her natural charm as well as her physical attributes. The twenty-first century cult burlesque artist Dita von Teese has drawn heavily on the style of Bettie Page for her look, and I have referenced her on a number of occasions. This is a very distinct look, with glossy black hair and a rollered fringe, with a pale, rosy complexion and scarlet lips.

Make-up

● Use a light-reflective concealer under your eyes and to even out any blemishes or uneven skin tone. Next, apply a creamy matte foundation, being careful to ensure a smooth, even finish.

● Groom eyebrows so they are neatly tapered, and define with a brow pencil if they're pale.

● Use a dark pewter-coloured shadow or eye pencil to create a smudgy, smoky look on the eyelids, with a fine line of black liquid liner close to the lashes.

● Use curlers to enhance your lashes, then apply individual false lashes to the outer corner of each eye, to give a natural-looking, longer-lash effect. Finish with two coats of black mascara.

● Use a peachy-pink powder blush to add a hint of natural rosy colour to the apple of the cheeks.

● Lips should be as near to a true bright red as possible, ensuring the shade is the correct one for your skin tone. Try a number of different reds to see whether you suit a slight blue tint or an orange tint – you'll be surprised at how many different shades of red there are, and it's worth persevering, because there's one to suit most women.

● Use a lipliner to create a smooth, full lip shape and paint on your chosen lip colour with a lip brush. Blot with a single ply of tissue, apply a dusting of loose powder, then repeat the process for maximum staying power. For a truly glamorous look, add some translucent gloss.

Hair

● Depending on the length of your hair, and how exaggerated you want the results to be, use the largest heated roller you can find to set your fringe, together with some setting lotion.

● Use large rollers in the rest of your hair, setting it into sleek waves that can be brushed out or swept into a ponytail.

Get the look

This is the era of legendary Hollywood pin-ups such as Marilyn Monroe, Brigitte Bardot, Jayne Mansfield and Elizabeth Taylor. I love the way these women looked: they oozed glamour from every pore, revelling in their curves, delighting in their femininity, and enjoying being worshipped by virtually every man on the planet.

Women such as Claudia Schiffer, Liv Tyler and Scarlett Johansson all interpret the 1950s look beautifully for the twenty-first century, and I regularly look to the Tinseltown pin-ups of the 1950s when I'm putting my own look together.

There are various versions of this look: the classic Marilyn make-up with red lips and lined eyes, the pale-lipped pout and smoky eyes of Brigitte Bardot and the classical elegance of Elizabeth Taylor, which is really a toned-down version of Marilyn's make-up. Here's how to recreate the different styles.

The Marilyn look

Although Marilyn Monroe was a peroxide blonde, this classic glamour make-up will suit different colourings too. It's what I describe as true pin-up make-up, and with a little practice it can be achieved with ease.

Make-up
● An even, natural complexion is the key to this look, as it's really about highlighting the primal sexual signals in the face, so a peachy skin with a rosy glow is what you're trying to achieve. To find the perfect blush colour, pinch your cheeks and look for a shade close to your natural blush.

● Sweep the eyelids and brow socket with a pale bone-coloured matte or slightly shimmery powder shadow. Then carefully apply a neat winged line of black eyeliner.

● Use curlers to enhance your lashes, then apply individual false lashes to the outer corners of the eyes to make your lashes appear longer. Finish with two coats of black mascara.

● Lips should be as near to a true bright red as possible, ensuring the shade is the correct one for your skin tone. Use a lipliner to create a smooth, full lip shape, and paint on your chosen lip colour using a lip brush. Blot with a single ply of tissue, apply a dusting of loose powder, then repeat the process for maximum staying power. Translucent gloss will up the glamour of this look.

Hair
● First of all, don't wash your hair for at least a day (I discovered early in my modelling career that hairdressers complained that my hair was too clean) as it is easier to style that way.

● You'll need some large heated rollers, some leave-in setting spray and time to get ready. Section your hair into two-inch chunks, spray lightly from the roots with the lotion and wrap smoothly around the heated rollers, ensuring the ends are tucked in neatly. After half an hour (or longer if possible), carefully unravel the curls and tease into shape using your fingers or a tail comb.

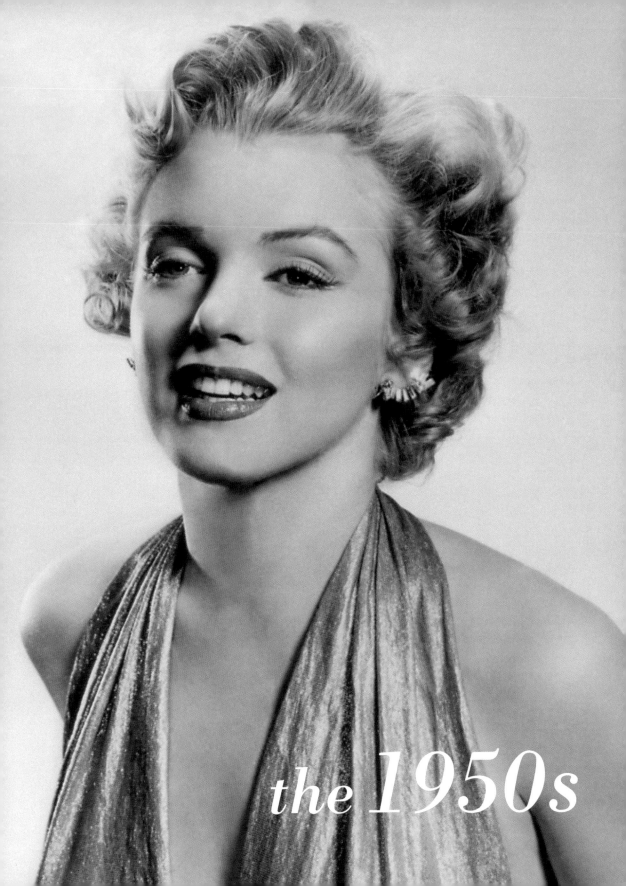

the 1950s

The Brigitte Bardot look

Combining the wide-eyed innocent look with the pale, perfect pout of a sex kitten is the key to this sultry style: the ingénue.

Make-up

● A dewy, natural-looking complexion is important – use a concealer and a light foundation if necessary.

● Soft pink or peachy blush should be swept onto the cheeks, temples, chin, and a little on the nose for a sunkissed, healthy glow.

● Eyelids and the brow socket should be swept with a biscuit-coloured matte powder shadow, with a deeper bitter chocolate blended into the crease to add contouring. Next, carefully apply a neat winged line of black eyeliner or use a damp brush to apply powder eye shadow in the same way on the upper lash line. Some people prefer to use shades of grey for a more smoky effect – it's all down to personal preference and your natural colouring, really. It's important to use the shades and textures that suit you – don't be dictated to by others.

● Use curlers to enhance your lashes, then apply individual false lashes to the outer corners of the eyes and towards the centre of the upper lid to give a natural, longer-lash effect. Use two coats of black mascara.

right: My hairstyle for the *Deuce Bigalow* premiere was inspired by Brigitte Bardot.

opposite: Brigitte Bardot works on the tousled, just-got-out-of-bed look.

● Use a light, tawny lip pencil to line the lips, and fill in using a creamy, fleshy pink lip colour. Blot and reapply.

Hair

Use your largest rollers to add some volume, back-combing a little if necessary, and shake out for a tousled, just-got-out-of-bed look that's natural and very sexy. .

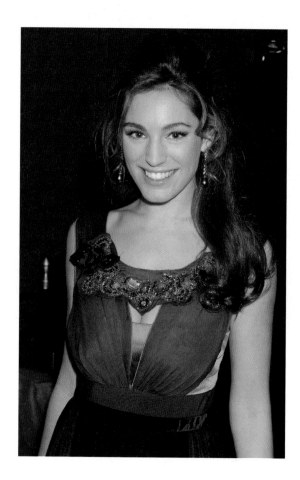

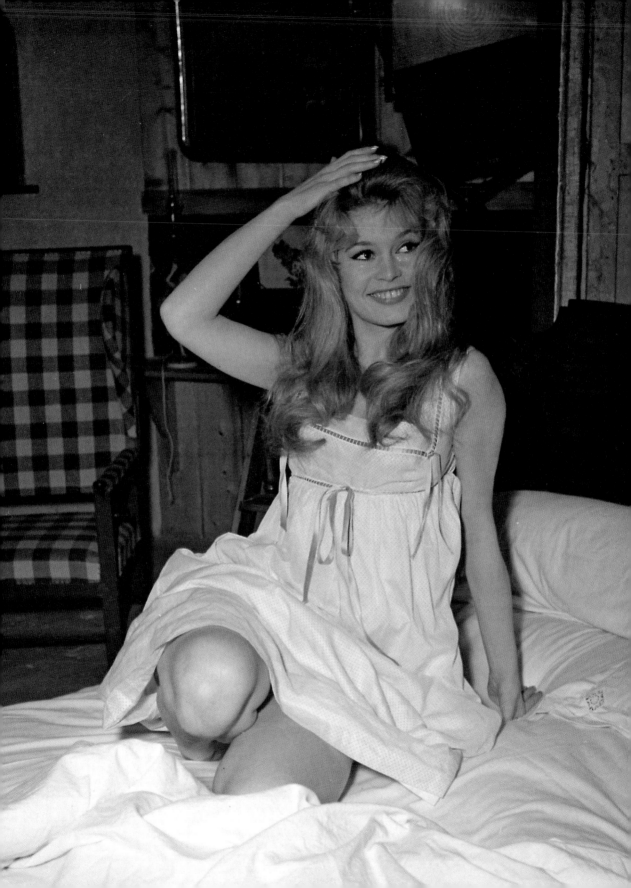

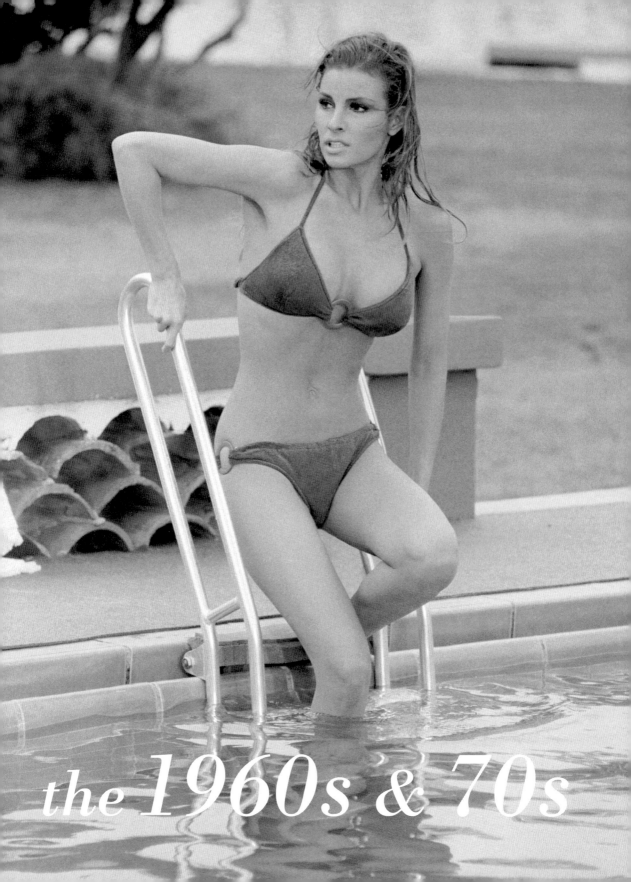

the 1960s & 70s

Get the look

Raquel Welch epitomises everything I love about this era: newly liberated women discovering their sexual prowess and playing with their image. As the Seventies dawned, Welch and her contemporaries were fabulous role models for a whole generation of women with their self-confident approach to female allure. In contrast to the bra-burning feminists of the time, Welch exuded a new female empowerment that celebrated womanhood, revelling in the delights of her body, face and gorgeous mane of hair.

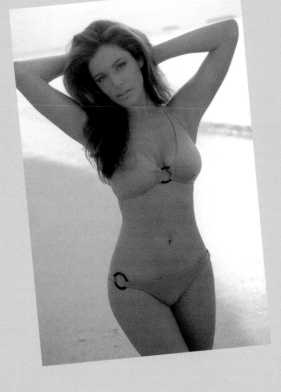

Make-up

● For the first time in history – although Brigitte Bardot did sunbathe, she was never particularly tanned – golden, sunkissed skin was fashionable, So after using a dab of concealer where necessary, and a sheer foundation, apply tinted moisturiser for a dewy, golden glow.

● Using a large brush, first tapping on the side of a basin to shake off excess powder, dust bronzing powder over the cheeks, nose, forehead and chin – it's best to start with a light application and add more as necessary.

● Use a shimmery pale gold eyeshadow in the brow socket and a bronze colour on the lid and in the crease of the eye. Apply a dark brown liquid liner to the upper lash line and, after using eyelash curlers, apply two coats of dark brown or black mascara.

● After lining the lips with a tawny pencil, use a creamy-textured tawny-pink lipstick to create a neutral, sexy pout.

Hair

Use the largest rollers you have to add some volume, backcomb a little if necessary and shake out for a tousled, bed-head look that's natural and very sexy.

left and above: Raquel Welch epitomised a new concept of feminine empowerment in the Seventies, and it is a look I adore creating.

Kelly's great hair guide ^㉑

I've always had long hair, so it's especially important to ensure it's in tip-top condition. There's nothing worse than long locks that are split and dry at the ends, as you lose all the lusciousness and impact a great mane should have.

I can't stress enough the importance of a *fabulous* haircut. So many women skimp on their hair, but are happy to splash out on shoes, make-up and clothes that linger unworn in their wardrobes. Your hair is the one accessory you carry with you *every* day of your life, so make it the one that you invest in. Forget an expensive bag, if your hair is well cut, in a way that suits your face shape, hair type and lifestyle, you will feel so much more confident when you leave the house in the morning.

You know how a bad hair day drags you down? Well, imagine how great you'd feel if every day was a good hair day? Your hairdresser should be someone who really respects and understands you and your needs: it's no good them using you as a guinea pig so they can experiment with the latest catwalk look. They need to know about your lifestyle: how much time you're prepared to spend on your hair each morning, how often you wash it – do you shower in the morning, then again at the gym after work? – how capable you are of blow-drying, and all the other factors relevant to daily maintenance. If they're not prepared to listen and adapt their approach to suit your needs, offering their experience and expertise to develop the best style for you, find another hairdresser.

That's not to say you should always get the cut you want: if you walk into the salon demanding to have hair like Jemima Khan, and your hairdresser suggests that your fine, fragile locks cannot be transformed thus; listen. Likewise, if you show him or her a picture of a sleek, streamlined bob, and are told it will be high maintenance, involving daily blow-drying of your naturally wavy hair, don't complain when it looks like a limp, curly mop because you can't be bothered with the effort. Always remember that the styles you see on the beauty and fashion pages of magazines have taken hours of effort – likewise those on celebrities on the red carpet. No one walks around looking like they've stepped out of a fashion shoot – not even the supermodels. Be realistic about what's achievable and work with what nature has given you, not against it.

right: Modelling classic Fifties-style hair at the British Fashion Awards in 2006.

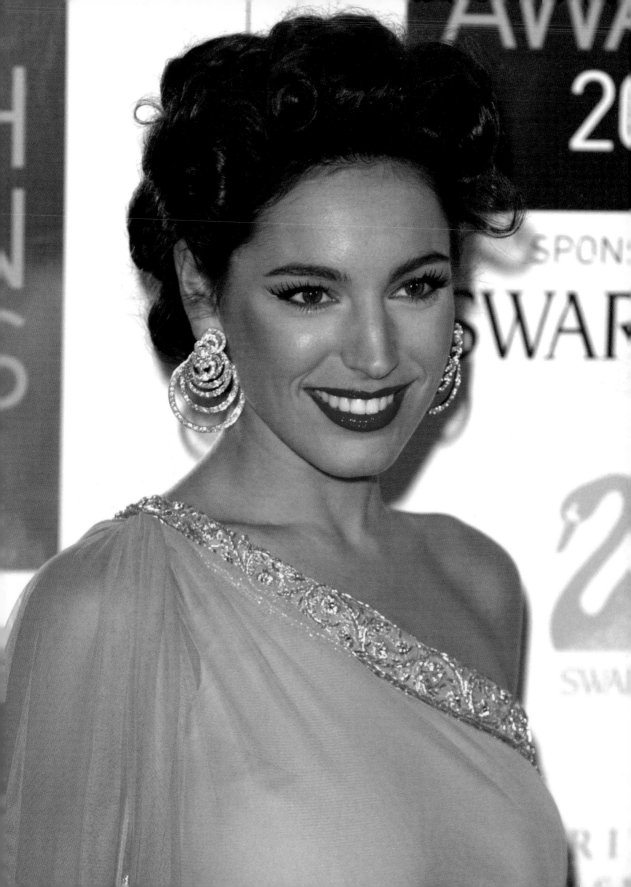

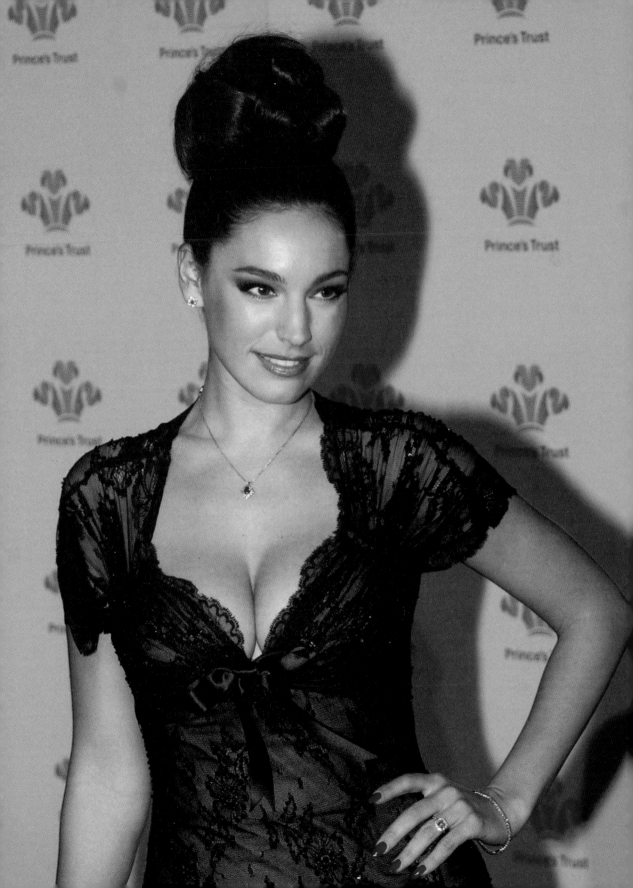

Consider the dimensions of your face and the proportions of your body when deciding on a style: petite, elfin women can be swamped by a massive mane of hair, while an overly bouffant bob can serve to emphasise an already round face. Hair is not only an extension of your style, but also your personality. If you're naturally reserved and like to blend in, don't go for an attention-grabbing colour, for example.

Good hairstyles come about because of a collaboration between stylist and client. If your stylist makes you feel like they're doing you're a favour by cutting your hair, dump them: you are the customer. If you can develop a strong, mutually respectful relationship with your hairdresser, I promise you'll benefit in the long term.

Once you've found a style to suit – and don't forget, you should evolve your look as time passes: what suited you at twenty may not look so great at thirty or forty, say – here are my tips on maintaining fabulous hair:

● It's important to have regular trims, so that the ends of your hair remain in good condition. There's no point in hanging on to an extra inch if it's damaged and split – that's not hair, that's baggage.

● Use a deep conditioning treatment once every three to six weeks, depending on the state of your hair. Head massage is more than just a nice sensation: it stimulates the nerve endings and blood circulation around the hair follicles, encouraging healthy hair growth.

● I try hard not to blow-dry my hair more than is necessary, as regular over-heating can be drying and damaging. If I'm on a modelling assignment or going out to a function, of course I blow-dry my hair – there's no doubt that if you're trying to create a proper 'do', you need heat to control your style – and you can't beat the skill that a really good hairdresser brings to blow-drying and styling hair. They can make the difference between a good 'do' and a fabulous one. But on a day-to-day basis, I simply shampoo with a gentle, neutral pH product, condition, blot dry with a towel – never rub as this can damage the cuticle, or protective outer layer, of the hair – and leave my hair to dry naturally.

● When it comes to looking after your hair, I believe in investing in good quality tools and products. Although the initial outlay may seem high, if you look after them, they'll last you a lifetime.

● I use a natural bristle hairbrush by Mason Pearson – every hairdresser I have ever worked with recommends these – as they're gentle on the hair and scalp. A good hairdryer will have a number of different speed and heat settings, so you can use cool air to help set the hair after drying, and a low speed on higher heat so you don't blast your hair with overpowering high temperatures. If you're using straightening irons, for example, use steam ones rather than ordinary heated ones, and buy the kind that have ceramic plates rather than metal, as they are gentler on your hair.

left: An elegant up-do can transform your look. Here I am at the Prince's Trust Gala Evening.

● Use non-chemical vegetable dyes on your hair. This is what I use to subtly alter my hair colour throughout the year. I don't like to use harsh chemicals and bleach, so Daniel Galvin Jnr, who has been colouring my hair for over a decade, uses organic colours to enhance the natural tones of my hair at different times of the year, reflecting and enhancing the way it changes naturally with exposure to the sun.

In the autumn, I tend to add reddish, auburn low-lights, and then a darker, deep brunette in winter to flatter my paler complexion. In the spring, I'll go for a golden, mid-brown, and in the summer, my hair will be a honey-blonde, all in tune with my natural skin tone throughout the year. Because I make these changes gradually as the months pass, they don't seem too dramatic, but if you compared a photograph of me taken in December with another taken in June, you'd probably see a huge contrast in the way I look.

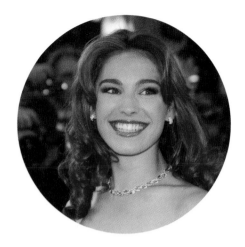

● Don't be afraid to use hairpieces if you want to create an amazing coiffure for a special night out. I don't generally need to, because I have very thick hair, but if you have fine hair, or just want to add more volume, do what loads of celebrities and models do, add a temporary hair piece. You can get different sorts, and good ones really do blend in seamlessly with your natural locks. I don't think hair extensions are a great idea long term: whether they're woven or glued in, you're damaging the roots of your natural hair, which are extremely fragile. I've seen lots of people with bald patches as a result of prolonged use of extensions. It's far better to get a great cut that accommodates your hair type and lifestyle on a day-to-day basis, then add a hairpiece if you want to for a big occasion.

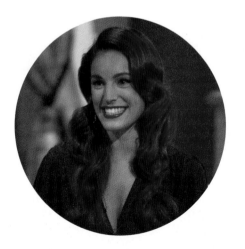

right: Going blonde for the summer in Cannes.

left: With reddish, auburn hair while being interviewed by Sharon Osbourne.

above: I tend to wear my hair a light brown colour in the spring.

● Hair accessories aren't just for children: I love using stretchy hair bands, head scarves and flower pins to create different looks. Inspired by my favourite style icons, I sometimes use the kind of elastic hair bands ballet dancers wear, like Brigitte Bardot, Natalie Wood and other glamorous stars. You can also use a rolled or folded silk twill headscarf in this way, which looks very chic.

● I also love to use fresh flowers or silk corsage blooms in my hair – added to a ponytail band or pinned just above the ear, they can look really glamorous and add a splash of feminine colour to your style.

● Although modern technology should be utilised because it's generally more advanced in terms of caring for your hair, i.e using gentle products as opposed to harsh chemicals, I do think some traditional techniques have a value. I don't understand why more women don't use their hairdresser for a regular set, like our mothers used to do. Nowadays 'setting' your hair is much softer and less uptight, and spending half an hour in the salon having your hair rollered and set means you don't have to worry about your hair looking good for at least a week. I regularly have my hair set, because I love the glamorous end result and the fact that it's so low maintenance afterwards. It just proves the point that doing the so-called 'fashionable' thing isn't always the most glamorous or flattering option. I'd rather have classically set womanly hair than the latest razor-cut bob any day of the week!

235

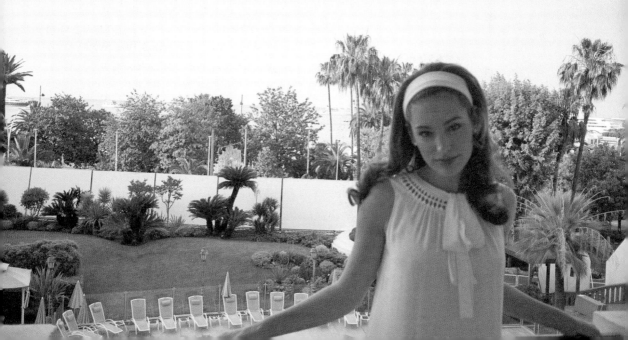

conclusion

So, here we are... You've read about my style icons and how I've used them to inspire a complete 'look' to suit my body shape and lifestyle. Now, it's your turn to find the pin-up that you most admire and pin down the pin-up within you...

I hope that, having read through the chapters of this book, you will have the confidence to experiment a little with your own personal style, and start a journey towards identifying an image that works for you. As I've said on a number of occasions within the pages of this book, it's not about mimicking a celebrity's wardrobe, or turning yourself into some 1950s parody, but about using the glamour of those who inspire you to inject a little starlet style into your own life.

I suggest you start by compiling your own scrapbook (either a proper, big, glue-pictures-on-the-pages number like you had at school, or a folder in which you keep picture references on your computer, say) to record all the images you like in one place. The internet is a wonderful resource when you are researching Hollywood icons and their style: I've become addicted to search engines that throw up a proliferation of photos and illustrations that I've never seen before. Once you start to collate postcards, magazine tear-sheets and suchlike, you'll be surprised how quickly you start to build a 'look-book', which can be the foundation of your new style.

As you gather images, look for the constants that seem to appear throughout: maybe the style you admire is all about a certain silhouette, or wearing stack-heeled shoes, for example, then start looking for those shapes when you're out shopping. Don't pressure yourself if it doesn't work to start with: if you're not comfortable in something, you're not going to feel good and then you certainly won't look gorgeous and glamorous.

Don't forget, this isn't about trends and having this season's must-have item, but sometimes fashion will swing your way and you'll find the catwalks and the high street are bursting with 1940s pencil skirts or 1950s dirndl skirts for example. If that's the look you have found works for you, then snap things up when they're available. Other times, you'll find yourself exasperated because there's nothing in the shops that seems to fit with your style. That's when it's worth trawling vintage stores, or maybe even making friends with a good dressmaker who can use your choice of fabric to make up sewing patterns to suit you.

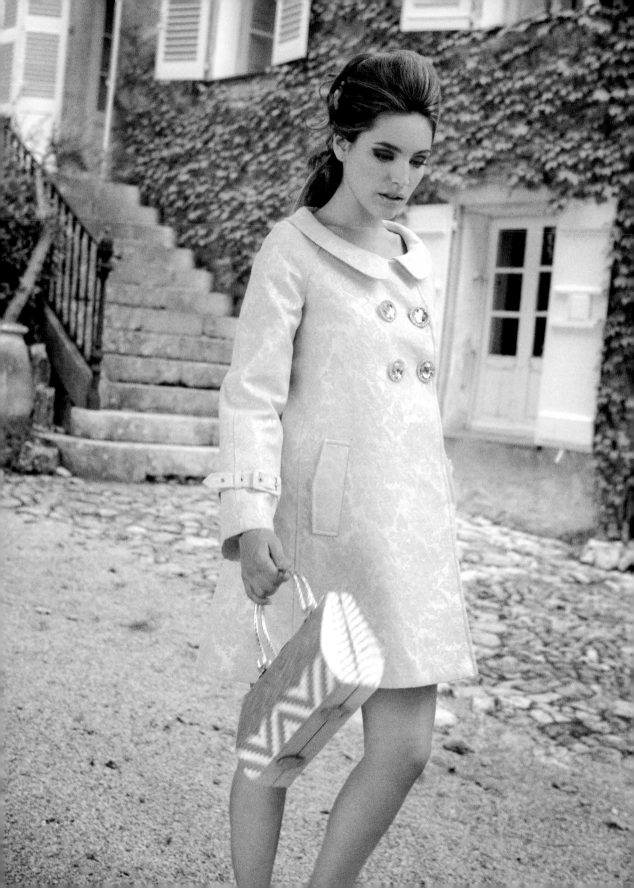

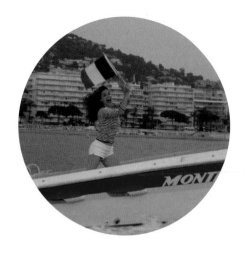

left: An off-duty moment during the shoot for this book.

Take time out to experiment with hair and make-up, too. Sometimes, all you need is a bit of expert advice from a great professional who can guide you towards a new hair cut, or a different way of blow-drying your existing style. Most good hairdressers offer free consultations and if you take your 'look book', they'll tell you what's achievable to suit your hair type, face shape and lifestyle (there's no point going for a high maintenance style if you are a working mother of three who barely has time to clean her teeth in the morning, for example). The same goes for cosmetics: one of the best investments you can make is a professional make-up lesson from someone who's not trying to sell a particular product. They'll teach you all the techniques to get really polished looks that are flattering, and give unbiased advice on which products are best to create the look you're after.

Most of all, though, what I really want to do is to reiterate that fashion is fun. For me, playing with clothes and my image is a way to enjoy toying with the way I present myself to the world. I don't take it too seriously, and it's all a big game of dress-up. What's really important to remember is that if you are happy, you'll look great, and forcing yourself to confirm to a certain code of dressing isn't going to make anyone happy.

So, girls, start collecting pictures for your look-book, and have some fun with your wardrobe. Roll out the red carpet and pin down the pin-up within you!

picture credits

Daily Telegraph: 105

Daniela Federici: 215

David Wright: 145

Dean Freeman: 3, 8, 10-11, 14-15, 16, 24, 28, 30, 39, 58, 96, 106, 110-11, 140, 141, 147, 150, 162, 169, 172, 197, 198, 202, 207, 212, 217, 237, 240

Getty Images: 77, 102, 113, 117, 118, 120-21, 123, 124, 127, 130, 131, 154, 165, 167, 175, 180-81, 221, 222, 223, 226, 228, 232, 234

Heat magazine: 53

Ipso Facto Films/Stephen Morley: 74, 75

ITN source/Channel 4: 56-57

ITV plc: 88

James White/Corbis Outline: 84

Jack Guy/Corbis Outline: 184

Kelly Brook: 17, 18-19, 20, 22, 23, 25, 26, 34, 35, 36, 37, 38, 70, 72-3, 73, 76, 81, 82, 83, 90, 91, 93, 94, 95,108-9,188, 189, 190, 195, 200, 201, 203, 204, 205, 206, 210, 235, 238

Mike Golsby: 40, 173

MTV: 63

Medway Standard: 27

Merlin Enabnit: 144

PA Photos: 50, 55, 137, 178, 231

Peter Singh, Wire Images, Getty Images: 100-01

Popstar Pictures: 92

Rex Features: 32, 33, 79, 80, 89, 133, 134, 138, 143, 176, 179, 225, 227, 234

Rankin: 153

Simon Emmett: 99

The Foto Factory: 42

Universal Pictures: 68

Warner Bros. Entertainment Inc: 71

Willy Camden: 87

Special thanks to Celebrity Pictures who provided the following photos:
45, 46, 64, 65, 67, 78, 81, 114, 135, 157, 158, 161, 167, 183, 187, 191, 192, 229

Orion Books would like to thank everyone involved in the production of the photo shoot, especially Dean Freeman, Richard Poulton and Polly Banks. Thanks also to Figleaves and Paul & Joe for their contributions.

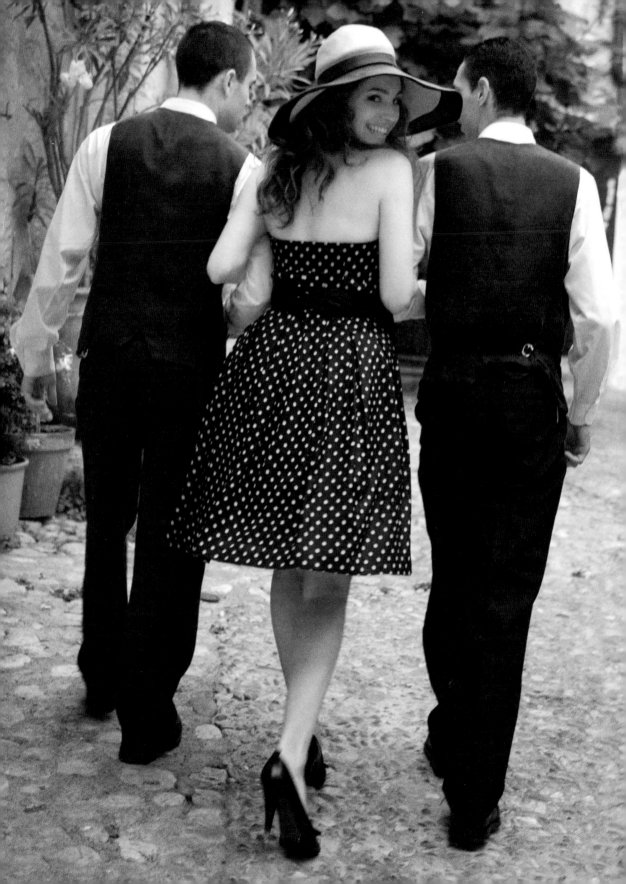

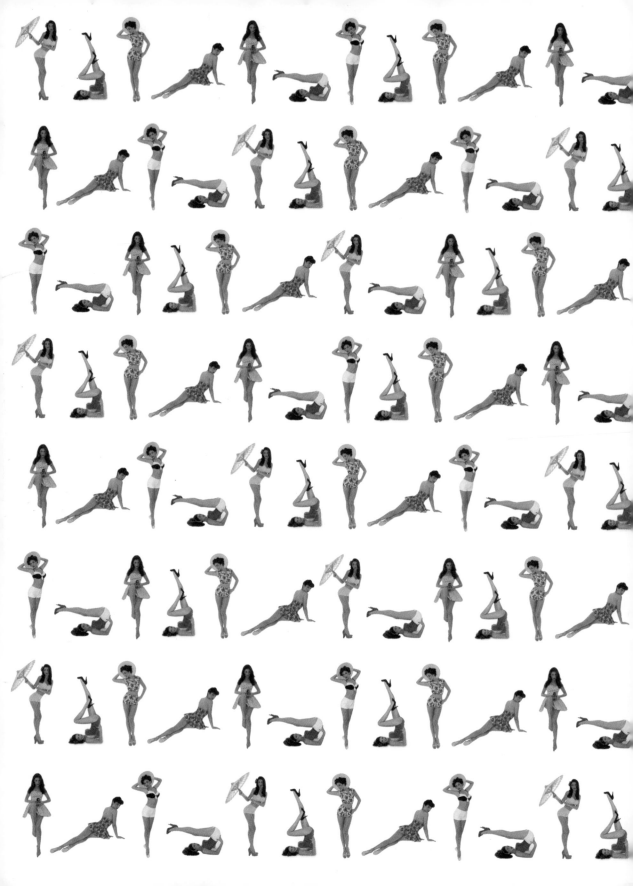